What oth
Healthcare and the Mission of God

"Dr. Paul Hudson is a healer. I mean that in every sense of the word. He's a doctor, concerned not only with healing the diseased and also promoting health in people and communities. In his long career, he's also been an effective mission leader, concerned with healing hearts and lives broken by sin while promoting gospel flourishing in people and communities. In this book, beautifully written and well-researched, he offers a prescription for an unfortunate wound: the sad fracture of Word-based evangelism from deed-based medical care. Paul argues convincingly for a holistic gospel proclaiming healing/salvation for whole persons and the whole cosmos. Only such a Word and Deed approach to redemption will reflect the gospel of a Messiah who came both preaching and healing the sick, the lame and the blind. Take up this book; engage its heart-gripping stories, and wrestle with his argument. It's a healing balm for your soul!"

John R. Sittema, pastor, author of *Meeting Jesus at the Feast*

"This helpful book, written from the perspective of more than three decades of medical missions experience and leadership, is an indispensable guide for those interested in understanding cross-cultural medical ministry and joyfully aligning healthcare professions with God's purposes in our broken world. I just wish this book had been available when I started my medical missions career 40 years ago."

Tim Teusink, MD, MA (Bioethics)

"This profound and practical book will be transformative to those planning to be medical missionaries or those already serving overseas. It shares the best antidote to burnout. It contains a prescription that will give you strength and joy as you face overwhelming needs. It provides a vaccine against disillusionment and much more. It is a 'must' read!"

David Stevens, MD, MA (Ethics); CEO Emeritus of the Christian Medical & Dental Associations (USA)

"An excellent resource and must-read for all those who are in or interested in health and healing. It holds together theology, praxis, life stories, and experiences very well."

Mathew Santhosh Thomas, MD, Training Coordinator and Regional Secretary (South Asia), International Christian Medical and Dental Society

"Dr. Paul Hudson is the most missiologically astute physician I have ever known. His medical education is certainly top drawer (two degrees from Johns Hopkins), but his missional experience may top even that. He has served both medically and in mission leadership roles for over three decades in Ethiopia, Thailand, and Nepal, not to mention leadership in national (USA) and international professional societies and task forces to address challenges such as HIV and AIDS in Africa. The volume you are holding is a labor of love from a godly man of vision who desires that medical missions should be all that it can be in providing excellent medical care, and in discipling the nations in the name of Jesus. No healthcare worker or mission leader who loves the Lord should miss reading this book."

Gary Corwin, missiologist, author, and editor, EMQ and *By Prayer to the Nations: A Short History of SIM*. Co-author of *Introducing World Missions: A Biblical, Historical, and Practical Survey*

"This book is written from—and with—a burning heart by a seasoned medical missionary who is passionate about making readers 'see the beauty of this calling' without neglecting the odds and frustrations faced in such a ministry. Hudson not only shares personal experiences and struggles in an honest, truly humbly manner. He relates all such experiences and his medical activities to the greater story of God as narrated in scripture. His wise counsel is discerning and reflective and, thus, it certainly will be of immense value for all those contemplating to engage in Christian healthcare missions near and far in one way or the other."

Christoffer Grundmann, author of *Sent to Heal! Emergence and Development of Medical Missions*

"This rare gem brings together wonderful stories, astute theological insights, honest self-critique, and integrative wisdom that will both inspire and create a solid foundation for those called to follow Christ in the healing of the nations. With a keen understanding of our human limitations, a trust in the power of God to accomplish his mission, an insightful exegesis of scripture, and a synthesis of pearls of wisdom of those who have gone before us, Dr. Hudson weaves a narrative that is both personal and transformational for a new generation. Having worked with Dr. Hudson to co-design and co-teach the Christian Global Health in Perspective Course, I am thrilled to see his time-tested and thoughtful insights bottled up like a well-crafted ship in a bottle, and I pray with him that this bottle lands on every shore and in every heart longing for God's healing presence."

Daniel O'Neill, MD, MTh, Managing Editor, Christian Journal for Global Health, co-editor and author of *All Creation Groans: Toward a Theology of Disease and Global Health*

"Paul's book gives a helpful reflection on the development of healthcare mission, especially in cross-cultural work. He has an easy-to-access style, with helpful questions to stimulate personal reflection and response. I highly recommend it to those who are on a journey into global health and mission."

Fi McLachlan, Head of CMF Global, UK

"Dr. David Livingstone, probably the most famous missionary of the 19th century, explained his work in Africa by noting that "God had an only Son, and he was a missionary and a physician." In his important book *Healthcare and the Mission of God*, Dr. Paul Hudson captures not only the theological truth of Livingstone's insight but also the practical reality. Dr. Hudson has done a masterful job of not separating what God has joined together: body and soul, faith and reason, religion and science, ministry and medicine. Not only does his book emphasize the importance of understanding the mission. It also underscores the importance of understanding the missionary."

Stan Key, Minister at Large. OneWay Ministries

"This book by Dr. Paul Hudson speaks deeply to the mind, body, and soul. With thirty years of medical missionary experience in three countries, Paul speaks candidly as one wounded but healed and who is committed to ministering to the whole person. Through moving personal stories, Paul explains how Christian healthcare ministry is motivated by the Bible's whole story and God's whole work in restoring our broken world. The gospel is both spoken and seen, as demonstrated in healthcare ministry, which integrates the cultural and evangelistic mandates. We are called both to be disciples of Christ and to make disciples of Christ, locally and cross-culturally. This book answers the question, 'Where does my little life fit into the grand story of God's mission?'"

Dr. Patrick Fong, Global Ambassador, OMF International

"Dr. Paul Hudson has written a crucial book for cross-cultural medical workers based on his decades of service on 3 continents, from bedside doctor to mentor of physicians. He has been a profound encouragement in my journey. I would strongly encourage prospective and experienced cross cultural medical workers to read this book in order to understand better their purpose in building Jesus Christ's kingdom and to avoid making the mistakes of many previous generations."

Niles Batdorf, MD, missionary surgeon serving with SIM

"For 40 years, I have had the privilege of listening to, crying with, struggling alongside, and counseling healthcare missionaries. I have not found a book that addresses the person God calls to serve Him in healthcare mission so comprehensively and holistically. Dr. Hudson explores where and how we can find boundaries and balance to help us persevere joyfully in hard places through tough times. He describes how to achieve a sustainable ministry of personal faith, discipleship with others, and healthy perseverance. I will certainly be using this as a resource and recommending it to anyone engaging in God's mission with healthcare."

Jarrett W. Richardson III, MD, Psychiatrist, Rochester, MN
Former Chair Christian Medical and Dental Associations
CMDE Commission
Former Chair Board of World Missions,
Evangelical Covenant Church

HEALTHCARE AND THE MISSION OF GOD

Finding Joy in the Crucible of Ministry

Paul J. Hudson, MD

Copyright © 2024 Paul J. Hudson, MD

All rights reserved.

No part of this book may be reproduced, stored in a retrieval system, or transmitted by any means, electronic, mechanical, photocopying, recording, or otherwise, without written permission from the author except for the use of brief quotations.

ISBN (Paperback): 979-8-9904362-8-2
ISBN (eBook): 979-8-9904362-7-5

Library of Congress Control Number: 2024906918

Scripture taken, unless otherwise noted, from the *New American Standard Bible*, copyright 1960, 1962, 1963, 1968, 1971, 1972, 1973, 1975 by The Lockman Foundation. Used by permission.

https://pauljhudson.com

Cover design: Elisabeth Kvernen

Genesis Publishing
Tulsa, OK

As Moses lifted up the serpent in the wilderness, even so must the Son of Man be lifted up; so that whoever believes will in Him have eternal life.

John 3:14-15

Foreword

I first met Paul in late 1993 at a consultation in Kenya held to discuss our mission organization's community services. A few years later Paul visited Galmi Hospital in Niger where I and my wife, also a physician, were serving as medical missionaries sent from Nigeria. The aim of his trip was to discuss healthcare ministry strategy across Niger. Over the years, Paul and I have participated in consultations addressing HIV and AIDS and other community health and services projects across SIM's many countries. Later, after I became SIM's International Director in 2013, Paul took on the role of our mission's point person for health ministries globally. He and his capable team were a tremendous resource to me during both the Ebola epidemic of 2014 and the Covid pandemic several years later. Needless to say, over the past 30 years, Paul and I have spent countless hours as fellow physicians, mission workers, and leaders of health ministries.

We have both experienced the many sources of daily stress for medical workers, including the workload, scarcity of resources, staffing shortages and inadequate training, relationship challenges, leadership gaps, and local worldviews and practices that may contribute to illness. The world in which we live today is increasingly complex. Economic and political crises mean that security has become a significant issue in many of the places where medical missionaries are needed most. The pressures of the work continue to undermine the longevity, joy, and capacity to thrive for many medical missionaries. It is no surprise that these challenges can result in burnout and premature return from the place of ministry.

And yet, the main thing and the "why" of medical mission is the restoration of human beings to wholeness in their relationship with the living God (a vertical relationship) and with those around them (a horizontal relationship) and with themselves, their community and their environment (a circular relationship). It is to restore people to dignity and *shalom*, the fullness of which is only possible in Christ. The medical mission worker is a bearer of the good news of joy (Luke 1:14).

This book provides an excellent overview of the biblical basis for bringing *shalom* to individuals and their communities as well as the historical roots of medical ministry, reaching back to the early Church's radical practices of compassion towards the poor and sick in the pattern of Jesus. It continues through the founding of hospitals and over the centuries until the age of modern missions, including shifts in the last 50 years towards public health.

Medical missions remains one of the most impactful types of mission services, and perhaps one of the key openings into many communities that are otherwise closed or hostile to the gospel. Medical missions has repeatedly been shown to change attitudes to the gospel. Yet many missionaries do not thrive in their work, while others return home prematurely and burnt out. However, what if there were ways to equip the medical worker to flourish?

In this book readers will learn some of the mindset transformations that hold the key to reclaiming our true identities in Christ and functioning from a different paradigm in ministry. Such transformation is achieved only through the life-long journey of being a disciple and making disciples. Paul writes, "Making disciples is the core ministry goal of both healthcare ministry and mission. I pray you will grow in your passion for making disciples, not as a program but as a lifestyle."

With decades of experience in diverse cultures, and in the varied contexts of both hospital ministry and preventative community healthcare, Paul is a guide we can trust. He writes from the perspectives of a practitioner, mentor, consultant, and leader. I believe this book has the potential to inspire a generative discourse among mission healthcare workers, mission leaders, and church leaders, who must come together to understand the realities and collaboratively seek wise responses to the challenges, for the sake of both the lost and the called.

Paul's call to the reader to consider the ministry of leadership within the ministry of healthcare could not be more timely. Like the author, I am a mission physician who went on to serve in leadership roles. I believe that rightly oriented leaders are acutely needed – leaders of medical institutions, community health programs, and entire organizations – who can shepherd ministries towards a clearer vision of healthcare fully integrated with other ministries for God's Kingdom purposes.

Whether you are a medical professional or an informal church-based health worker, whether you are flourishing or struggling in your ministry, this practical book will help to ground you in the biblical and historical foundations of health ministry. It will also help you to avoid the false dichotomies of physical "versus" spiritual care, and it will refresh your vision and hope for the enormous capacity of health ministries to partner with the church for the growth and flourishing of the Kingdom everywhere.

Dr. Joshua Bogunjoko
SIM International Director, 2013-2024
Jan 16, 2024

Dedication

Clare, you are a loving wife and faithful helper.
I could not have done this book without you.
I am thankful to God for our journey together.
You are my treasure.

Contents

Foreword xi
Dedication xv
Introduction xix

Part I: Losing the Big Picture 1
Chapter 1   The Challenging Journey in
             Healthcare Missions.. 3
Chapter 2   Embracing Our Brokenness................................ 15

Part II: Discovering God's Purpose 29
Chapter 3   Created as Whole Persons,
             Created for Purpose 31
Chapter 4   Disease, Sin, and the Corruption of Purpose 47
Chapter 5   Health, Salvation,
             and Restoration of God's Purpose....................... 65
Chapter 6   Saving Bodies and Saving Souls 79

Part III: Aligning God's Purpose with Healthcare 95

Chapter 7	Healthcare Ministry and Making Disciples 97
Chapter 8	Church, Compassionate Care, and Culture 115
Chapter 9	Health, the Church, and the Mission of God 127
Chapter 10	Medical Missions and Healthcare Missions........................... 143

Part IV: Serving with God's Purpose...................................... 167

| Chapter 11 | Leadership in Healthcare Mission .... 169 |
| Chapter 12 | Following Christ's Call in Healthcare............... 185 |

Appendices 199

Appendix A	A Liturgy for Medical Providers 201
Appendix B	Recommended for Further Reading................. 205
Appendix C	Selected Definitions 217

Acknowledgements 223

Introduction

After more than thirty years of experience as a medical missionary in three countries, I have experienced both the joys and frustrations of medical mission service. I've had the privilege of helping fellow physicians and nurses align their efforts with the mission of God. I have also seen some of the pitfalls of ministry as a healthcare professional. I have faced (in myself and others) the tragedy of losing the path, being overwhelmed with work, and the pressure of the lack of resources.

Healthcare ministry can be a crucible – a vessel made to endure intense heat. A crucible tests and transforms its contents into something new. What if the crucible of ministry is also an invitation to joy? Jesus invites us as healthcare workers to be transformed with joy even as He works through us to heal others.

So, I am writing this book with a burden on my heart. I have felt the frustration of being overwhelmed trying to do healthcare and ministry together. I want to encourage others in the same work who may also be overwhelmed with fatigue, burnout, or confusion. As a physician, I am writing mainly for healthcare workers who serve or plan to serve in cross-cultural missions to the poor or marginalized.

Although I am an American, I hope that any modern healthcare provider around the globe will find something useful here. I am also an epidemiologist and believe that the gospel calls us to the healing of communities. This book may also help leaders responsible for integrating healthcare into their mission efforts.

I am writing to start a conversation, not simply about *what* we do but *why* we do it. Aligning healthcare ministry and the mission of God means aligning our purposes with God's. Healthcare involves care of individual patients as well as care for the community. I invite you to consider not just the activities of healthcare, but how these activities fit into God's plan for the world–the mission of God. It's easy to lose track of how our story fits into God's bigger story.

God's Word does not leave us in the dark about "why" we serve and how it impacts the building of His Kingdom. Scripture provides us with a clear narrative that integrates healthcare and the mission of God. Our modern culture and worldview distort that narrative, causing confusion and uncertainty about our role in that mission. We will see that healthcare can sometimes become an idol and overwhelm us by contending for God's place in our lives.

The rod of Asclepius is the image of the Greek god of healing and a symbol of rational medicine. We see the rod and serpent of Asclepius on everything from pharmaceutical products to medical society emblems. But the image of God's healing is a more ancient serpent, the one Moses raised onto a pole in the wilderness, foreshadowing the cross. (See Numbers 21:3-10). Medicine can become an idol, like the rod of Asclepius, if it captures our imagination apart from God. But, from the right perspective, it can lead us to the cross.

These pages will not only challenge our modern thinking about healthcare. They will also challenge our understanding of the gospel itself! Like one of my missionary colleagues, you may have experienced churches that see ministry to the body as a lure for the "real" ministry to the soul. Ministry to the body can become divorced from ministry to the soul, moving us away from God's purpose. We will discover that the Great Commission brings them together.

We must not allow healthcare to go in one direction while evangelism and church planting head off in another. Scripture gives us the foundation to integrate the whole person, body and soul. It also connects ministry to the individual with ministry to the community, including church planting. I believe God has given all that in the story of salvation, rightly understood.

Medical care of individuals has opened many hearts to the good news of salvation, as it demonstrates God's heart for the whole person. I saw this first very clearly as a young Christian and a medical student on a short-term mission trip in Kenya. My mentor, Dr. Bill Barnett, showed me how medical and spiritual conversations were natural partners. And while the hospital was the source of healing for many, it could not address root causes of illness, related to culture and poverty. But should the issues of culture and poverty be part of the agenda of healthcare or medical missions? We need God's perspective on the ministry of healthcare itself.

We will begin in **Part I (Losing the Big Picture)** with the story of my own medical mission journey in Ethiopia. In Chapter Two, we will meet other healthcare missionaries on their journeys. **Part II (Discovering God's Purpose)** will consider the broader story of what God has done in Christ, so Scripture becomes our framework for understanding healthcare and God's purpose (Chapters Three to Six). **Part III (Aligning God's Purpose with Healthcare)** will unpack the concept of "ministry," and how it relates to discipleship and the church. Ministries of compassion through the church throughout history have shaped the world (Chapters Seven and Eight). Chapter Nine will highlight the concept of "mission" and how healthcare ministry aligns with mission, the broader story of the work of God in the world. In Chapter Ten, we will look at ways this alignment of ministry and mission has been challenged over the past two centuries of medical missions. In **Part IV (Serving with God's Purpose)** we will consider leadership, with the prayer that the Lord will continue to raise leaders who will enable the church to better reach out to the world's suffering with the gospel.

By necessity, this book is a very brief starter. Please take it as an appetizer, raising issues and asking questions to discuss further with medical colleagues and mission leadership.

While your journey will not be the same as mine, I hope that by reading this book you will:

- Gain a clearer picture of healthcare ministry to people in need.
- Discover that healthcare and God's mission are not driven by separate agendas but flow from an integrated center, the heart of Jesus.
- Understand the importance of defining success by biblical values rather than cultural notions.
- See how the ministry of healthcare integrates with the Great Commission.
- Appreciate how to respond when the healthcare ministry itself is broken.

- Develop a closer walk with Jesus Christ and love for sharing the good news of salvation.
- Experience more confidence and less anxiety in ministry.
- Find hope and joy restored through better work boundaries, and thus experience less burnout and frustration.

My prayer is that the whole enterprise of medical missions (or healthcare missions) will be reinvigorated. Jesus cares about the suffering of this world, especially among the poor, marginalized, or oppressed. Christians around the globe are increasingly involved in healthcare ministry to address that suffering. Jesus is advancing His Kingdom through disciples renewed by a better grasp of the integration of healthcare and the gospel.

If you are not a follower of Jesus, I'd like to invite you to consider how the story of God's work in history might provide purpose for your own life and service in healthcare. I am so grateful for what I have learned from the Lord through many believers in Ethiopia, Nepal, and Thailand over the past three decades. I look forward to sharing some of my story with you. I trust this will connect with your story and ultimately with God's.

So, what is your story? Do you feel overwhelmed by the needs in your area? Are you frustrated by broken systems that prevent you from helping people? Are you feeling burned out? I know what that's like. All these challenges are maddening and can cause us to lose hope, even as we do our best to serve and obey God. In these pages, I pray you will find a safe place to sort out your frustrations and pain as we take a fresh look at our loving God and His plan for the nations—and for us.

PART I

Losing the Big Picture

CHAPTER 1

The Challenging Journey in Healthcare Missions

The tires on my Land Cruiser kicked up dust and gravel as I roared out the iron gates heading to the hospital in our town in southern Ethiopia. My wife, Clare, saw the commotion at the gate.

"What was that all about?" she asked me later that day.

"What do you mean?" I asked.

"Well, you are usually calm and collected. Are you mad? Frustrated? Is there something going on at work?" she replied.

My frustration was obvious to her but not to me. God used her comments to begin to stir my awareness. I was experiencing disappointment in ministry and a critical spirit. I felt all I was doing was just a drop in the ocean. My medical and mission training had not prepared me for the challenges I was facing. I was thrilled to be serving the Lord using medicine but felt overwhelmed and undervalued. I was not fun to be with.

From this beginning in Ethiopia, I discovered that the source of my frustration was not in my circumstances or performance, but in an unlikely place—myself! I struggled with unmet expectations. My ambitions were unrealistic. Although I didn't want to admit it at the time, I was angry that the changes needed were too daunting. I was frustrated with the work, the politics, and the culture. I wondered if the Lord had led us to the right place.

Our first overseas placement was in Ethiopia with SIM[1], a church-planting mission. The mid-1980s found my wife and me in Addis Ababa, green missionaries embarking on a year of formal Amharic language study before moving "down country" to the southernmost province bordering Kenya. In Arba Minch, the provincial capital, we hoped to come alongside our SIM-related churches, just emerging from a decade of communist oppression during which many believers had been imprisoned.

The local communist governor decreed we would not be permitted as foreigners to attend church services (it was hard to explain to the supporters at home that we didn't attend church on Sundays!). We were, however, allowed to meet for discipleship and prayer in our own home with local believers.

As an internist and epidemiologist, my official work permit was to provide support for the local Ministry of Health staff and practice clinical medicine in the local mission hospital. Unofficially, the mission understood I would work with local churches to address basic health needs in the community, such as better nutrition,

---

[1] SIM is an international, interdenominational mission called to make disciples of the Lord Jesus Christ in communities where He is least known. Our founders journeyed to difficult places to share the gospel since 1893. Today we serve on six continents and over 70 countries in multicultural teams. See https://www.sim.org/home

sanitation, and the treatment of simple problems. I was eager to see the church grow strong and be salt and light in its own community.

Longing for a wider impact

While I counted it a privilege to treat patients and even share my faith at the hospital, I wanted to see deeper changes in the community and culture, changes that would have prevented diseases in the first place. For example, traditional healers in the community commonly treated pharyngitis in children by cutting the uvula (the soft flap of tissue hanging down from the back roof of the mouth), which was often done with a dirty instrument. The sepsis which followed often ended in the child's death. Such tragedies could be prevented if behavior and culture were different.

At the same time, poverty, inadequate nutrition, and lack of access to healthcare contributed to disease mortality. Most of the families in the region lived far from modern healthcare, and women had nowhere to go for complicated labor. These systemic issues were entrenched in the culture since they went beyond individual behavior. The agreement SIM had with the government allowed me to address these sorts of community health problems, and I was eager to do it.

I hit the ground, ready to roll with a full toolbox of ideas. I had trained in international community health at Johns Hopkins under Dr. Carl Taylor, a pioneer in the field. I had also become an epidemiologist at the CDC in Atlanta and the State Health Department in Vermont, gaining practical "shoe-leather" approaches to the health of communities. In Ethiopia, I investigated community outbreaks, studied patterns of malnutrition and death in children, and trained health officers in disease control.

It may seem painfully obvious that I would not get far in changing behavior, but at that time, there was great enthusiasm for "Primary Health Care." WHO's Alma-Ata declaration in 1978 set a goal for global "health for all by the year 2000." It was the heyday of community or primary health, while hospitals were often accused of being "disease palaces," not making a community-wide impact. Mission organizations like SIM were getting on board with this focus on the community. My idealism went far beyond preventing disease. I learned about God's care for the poor in a Bible school course named "Theology of Poverty." I wanted to see communities move towards the *shalom* of God's Kingdom.

I believed the changes needed would come through believers and churches, so I spent time training and discipling believers. The Old Testament is clear about God's heart for the needy. "'He pled the cause of the afflicted and needy; then it was well. Is not that what it means to know Me?' declares the Lord."[2] I believed that God wanted his church to have a wider impact on Ethiopia. Ultimately, that meant changing culture, "the distinctive ideas, customs, social behavior, products, or way of life of a particular nation, society, people, or period."[3] In my case, it was the culture in and around Arba Minch, Ethiopia.

There were five local SIM-related house churches in our town. When we first arrived, the leaders asked us NOT to come to their house church meetings, since our presence would put believers at risk from communist authorities. For years, they had met secretly, if at all, singing quietly, leaving meetings separately; as a result,

---

[2] Jeremiah 22:16

[3] *Culture*, Oxford English Dictionary, https://www.oed.com/dictionary/culture_n?tab=factsheet#eid. (2023, September).

relationships among churches were few. Trust relationships among the house leaders were tenuous. As an outsider and newcomer, I slowly formed good relationships with these leaders, which led to invitations to preach or teach the Bible to their flock.

Despite building good relationships, however, I made little progress in moving the church toward meeting health needs in the community. I spent hours and days training believers, but there was little visible progress and seemingly little motivation for community change. Since churches were just beginning to meet after a decade of being scattered, priorities were on rebuilding basic trust and security and beginning to preach and baptize again. New initiatives in preventive health were definitely not on the top of their agenda. Despite all my efforts and training, I saw little progress.

Some believers told me that "development" work (like nutrition or healthcare) was a waste of time, like "throwing money into a river," compared to gospel preaching. Rather than reaching out to others, the church seemed embroiled in its own issues. While I was able to share the gospel with individuals, it seemed unlikely to make much impact. I believed God wanted to bring about changes in society through the church, and yet the church itself seemed resistant to change. What could I do to further God's Kingdom and righteousness on earth?

Dis-integration

My initial response to this dilemma was to work harder. Having successfully navigated multiple degrees and training programs, I was a high achiever. I had prepared for the more obvious challenges of medical missions, such as scarce resources, time limitations, tropical diseases, and a new language. With all this preparation, I thought I should have more answers than I had. I pushed myself hard, seeing patients in the hospital, training local public health workers, supervising nurses, and working in the community. I felt driven to meet the demands around me.

Despite all my efforts, I was frustrated by the task. Meeting the physical demands of medicine is tiring, but trying to change people and culture is overwhelming. I was unable to meet my own expectation of having all the right answers. My training and my efforts were not successful, and I didn't know why. I could only see the impossibility of the task. After several years of ministry, I grew discouraged and began to question my calling to medical missions. I even remarked to our U.S. mission director, "I am not sure I even believe in community health anymore!"

At the time, I did not understand that my driveness was a symptom of a deeper problem: my need to be valued and accepted. I wanted to be seen as competent, a good doctor, and a good missionary! In trying to change the world, I didn't see that the Lord first had to change me. Rather than rely on my own technical ability or competence, I had to first rely on His love and acceptance. He wouldn't allow me to proceed in my own strength.

In response to my ministry concerns, one of the Ethiopian Christian leaders, a dear brother in Christ and a pharmacist, said, "Dr. Paul, you must *think* but not *overthink*!" I laughed, but his words spoke the truth. Another Christian Ethiopian anthropologist helped to reset my expectations. I had told him, "It will take five years even to begin to know where to start to change the church and community." He replied, "It's worth it!" He repeated this three times during our conversation, knowing I was hoping for an easy way forward, not a slow, patient learning process. The Lord began to shape me through the faith of the Ethiopian people.

I began to learn that frustrations are normal. The path to ministry fruitfulness is often long and winding. Sometimes we feel stuck and must adjust expectations. Rather than blame my frustration on our mission leaders, church leaders, or government, I had to deal with my own blind spots, sin, and even idolatry. I was there for Jesus' ministry, not my own. I started to accept my own pride and idealism. I began to understand the Apostle Paul's admonition that God's grace is sufficient "for power is perfected in weakness." (2 Cor 12:9). Healthcare missions is a wonderful place to discover our weaknesses and blind spots!

I started to see, through the eyes of Ethiopian believers, that the foundation of my idealism was fractured. My understanding of cultural change and the Kingdom needed to mature. My assumptions about what "I" could do were self-oriented and prideful. I had to see the changes I needed in myself before I could change others. But God, by His grace, was patiently working in me.

Becoming a learner again

Although working with the church was frustrating, it was the believers in the church who helped me identify my unrealistic expectations and gave me hope. I had to learn in the crucible of ministry. Becoming a change agent in the world takes more than pre-field training. The patience of local believers and friends encouraged me to see how patient God is in changing us from the inside out.

The key to changing the world, I discovered, was not in my work or plans but in relationships. God, as Trinity, is relational, and He has made us for relationships. He heals us through relationships. It was through others that I began to experience healing. Gradually, I gained a perspective of God's sovereign control of everything—my circumstances, the ministry, my family—and my work towards His good purpose.

During our time in Ethiopia, I was able to disciple a group of six Christian young people who met with me weekly to discuss the Bible and health. Some were health professionals and some not. We encouraged one another as we considered what God's Word says about life, health, and salvation. Together, we dreamed of ways God could use the growing church to share the love of Christ with those suffering in communities around the churches.

One day, an Ethiopian evangelist visited our home in Arba Minch. We commiserated with each other over the lack of gospel witness in the hills surrounding us and the lack of unity in the house churches in our town. I shared some of my frustration with the church's inward focus. He said, "What are you doing next Tuesday? I'll come, and we will pray and fast for twenty-four hours." My first honest but silent reaction was to hope I had something else to do on Tuesday. I wanted to work *hard*, not sit and pray for a full day. But he and a friend did come. We alternated reading Scripture for an hour and then praying for an hour (in Amharic) all night. This was a new experience for me, but not for him!

Amazing! Within a week, the elders from the churches in town who had been in the conflict were confessing their sins to one another and begging for forgiveness. Forgiveness led to healing and God's blessings. Some time later, evangelists were sent to those hills with the gospel. Not only did the believers eventually establish new churches and a Bible school, but community health and HIV and AIDS ministries as well. It was the beginning of a work of God outward from the churches to communities in need.

Being disciples means being learners. Becoming learners again can be challenging, especially for those of us who already have impressive educations and a powerful drive to work hard. It is easy to assume we've "arrived" when we have become healthcare professionals. But I see now that we will never really "finish" learning from the Lord, especially during a challenging ministry. He makes us His disciples—His learners—by giving us people to learn from in the midst of ministry. We will discover that being and making disciples is fundamental to His purpose for us.

Handmade health ministry

Over the five years we spent in Ethiopia, my wife and I served faithfully but never saw many of the changes in the community that we dreamed of. Because of an escalating civil war, we were forced to leave the country in the spring of 1991. Yet, the churches continued to thrive and brought glory to God through Kingdom-transformed lives and communities. This progress became especially true after communism was toppled that same year. Today, the church denomination trains believers both in the Bible and in health, addressing the physical and spiritual needs of the district through hundreds of churches. Those churches today have gone far beyond what I could have done with my community health program, meeting both physical and spiritual needs. This initiative is helping to improve the health of the nation and even change the culture for God's glory.

The seeds planted in the original small group of trainees began to bear much fruit, too; some attended Bible school and years later matured to become regional and national leaders in the church. Our work was one small catalyst in a ministry that the Lord brought to fullness in His time. During that time of fullness, we were no longer living and working in Ethiopia.

I remain in awe that the Lord uses ordinary people like doctors and nurses to build His Kingdom and transform cultures. He uses us not because we are professionals, but because we trust Him. The blessings of the Kingdom are not based on *"our"* abilities but on God's love and faithfulness. We plan our activities, but His purposes will prevail.[4] When we are determined to trust Him, He delights to use us to demonstrate His character. Love is caught more than it is taught.

Frustrations and feelings of being overwhelmed are plentiful in cross-cultural healthcare missions. The Lord doesn't waste any of them. I hope you will begin to see that He has much in store for us to learn in the crucible of ministry, especially from local believers who know and understand the culture. God's mission is wide and glorious, as wide as His Kingdom; that wide and glorious mission begins with solid, Christ-honoring relationships. We have a small and important part to play, whether in the operating room or in homes in the community.

I traveled to a medical conference in Asia just after Clare and I had to leave Ethiopia. I found myself describing our experiences in Ethiopia to a Japanese physician I met on the plane.

"I don't know how many times I drank coffee with local believers, sharing Scripture and health principles," I explained. But change was not forthcoming. Despite my failings and shortcomings, the Lord heard our prayers. I told him the bigger story about how the Lord eventually used Ethiopian believers to bring about change.

---

[4] Proverbs 16:9

After a long pause, he mused, "Oh, I understand now, you are saying that community health is 'handmade'!" By this remark, he was saying that community health does not come from a program or set of activities, but by the hand of God working through our relationships. The

Frustrations and feelings of being overwhelmed are plentiful in cross-cultural healthcare, but the Lord doesn't waste any of them.

underlying rhythm of ministry is not mechanical but personal. I suggest that *all* healthcare ministries are "handmade." We have wonderful programs, some of which we use in a clinic or hospital and others in the community. But the Lord works personally with us in the midst of our programs and sometimes even without them. He sets the ministry pathway for us. Hebrews 12:1 tells us, "Let us run with endurance the race that is set before us." He personally sets the course for the race.

Healthcare mission does not stand alone but is part of a bigger design, *God's mission.* The mission of God is His work in the world, and in history, centered on God the Father, Son, and Holy Spirit. The mission of God can involve many different types of activities, like an orchestra with percussion, strings, and brass instruments. Christ calls us as healthcare professionals to join a symphony. The musical score is framed by Scripture, beginning with God's original design in creation and progressing to a new creation in Christ. We need to anchor healthcare ministry within this larger design.

As followers of Jesus Christ, we can expect to experience frustration and even suffering as we care for the health needs of others. I hope this book will help you put that suffering in the context of the mission of God in the world, giving it a larger perspective. It is important to see the value of our healthcare work; with Christ, the work has meaning in the light of His mission to make disciples of the nations.

My prayer is that God will use something of my own story to help you on your journey toward wholeness and integration, enabling you to connect your story to the larger story of God's work in the world.

Questions for reflection:

What is your story? What challenges have you found in your journey in healthcare ministry?

When does the ministry of healthcare feel broken to you? What is your inward response?

CHAPTER 2

Embracing Our Brokenness

Dr. Ethel Ambrose arrived in India from Australia in 1905 as part of the Poona and Indian Village Mission (now part of SIM). She worked hard at language and at meeting physical needs. But it was her character that her colleagues most appreciated. "Doctor's thoroughness and faithfulness begat the same in all who worked under her. Whatever had to be done was undertaken in a calm and thorough way. The harder she was pressed, the calmer she became—it was not that she did not feel things, for she had a fine sensitive nature, but God so ruled in her life that His grace was magnified in her. She was always first a missionary, then a doctor."[5]

There are many fine examples of doctors and healthcare professionals who have served the Lord as missionaries, but missionary biographies don't always reflect their struggles. We aspire to serve like Dr. Ambrose, as Christians who happen to be medical professionals rather than medical professionals who happen to be

---

[5] G.R. Corwin, *By Prayer to the Nations* (Credo Press, 1st Ed., 2018), 275.

Christians. But based on my experience, many of us struggle in the journey. In fact, one of the premises of this book is that struggle is normal. Like those we serve, we know something of our own brokenness and that of our families and communities. The point is not to allow struggles to defeat us but to heal us.

Let's look at the lives of three (fictional but realistic) healthcare missionaries to identify some of their struggles. Their stories highlight some of the distress that I encounter among healthcare workers.

Cindy

Cindy was called to be a missionary medical doctor as a child. She trained in general practice and rural medicine; this education helped her tremendously in her first years of service in a mission hospital in rural Botswana. She loved the Lord and appreciated being part of an organization that aimed to share the gospel. As a single person, she was devoted to her work and soon became the head of the medical staff. No one questioned her competence or dedication, but the stress of the work and the challenges of limited resources strained her. She became so caught up in the day-to-day busyness of the ministry that she was unaware of how her decisions affected others. Ministry was becoming more about her own efficiency and service than her love for others. She was not aware of the anger brewing inside, but she was aware that she was losing her joy.

Cindy became increasingly tired and had difficulty sleeping. At odds with nurses and doctors in the hospital, she began isolating herself emotionally. She was clearly headed for an emotional breakdown but had no idea how to avoid it while managing a busy hospital. The hospital CEO, a fellow doctor, was able to confront her before a full-blown burnout occurred.

"Cindy, you must stop! You can't continue like this," he said.

"What choice do I have? The needs are only increasing, and I may have to do a couple more on-calls this next week."

"You know you are in crisis, and I will not allow you to continue to go down. We are making a new plan!"

Cindy finally did yield to her boss's tough love. She didn't just take time off but went back to her home country, where her mission agency arranged counseling, rest, and coaching for her. She was surrounded by folks who helped her identify the source of her burnout and take steps toward healing. After several months, she was able to return to the field with more insight into her own needs, as well as a plan for better coping. She has already started to find more insight, clearer purpose, better boundaries, and more joy.

Like Cindy, the biblical character Martha found her purpose in serving others but was worried and distracted by the act of serving itself. She became resentful of Mary, who was focused on Jesus.[6] We, too, can get so caught up with the needs of the work that the needs themselves drive us. As healthcare workers, we are tempted to be the Savior rather than letting the Savior work through us.

The Lord rebuked Martha, not for her serving but for her loss of perspective. He showed her His purpose *in* and *beyond* serving. Mary found that purpose in loving Jesus and sitting at His feet. Martha had to choose to begin anew to work with more singleness of heart.

Despite our best intentions, we struggle to serve God *and* love our neighbors (patients, staff, and colleagues). We do many good things, but sometimes we find it hard to prioritize the best over the good. Some days are great and full of joy. But healthcare can

---

[6] Luke 10:38-42

take on a life of its own and begin to drain us. The needs around us are never-ending. Where do we find boundaries to keep us from overworking?

Like Cindy, we are tempted to meet external demands by working harder. Doctors, nurses, and health professionals are expected to fix things, and often we can do so, even in the face of impossible odds. In our desire for excellence, we often expect we can do the impossible. Ultimately, we are limited by our humanity. Healing does not come just by working harder.

A strong biblical foundation—and healthy relationships—will keep us from being enslaved by our own good works. We were made to work, yet this very good thing (work in healthcare) can defeat us. It defeated Cindy, not just because the external demands were so big, but also because she was not able to make clear boundaries for her work. Her work was not framed as much by God's purposes as by her own.

> **A strong biblical foundation—and healthy relationships—will keep us from being enslaved by our own good works.**

Ministry is fulfilling God's purposes through our work. If the purpose is unclear or lost, ministry can become *any* activity we do, often driven by forces within us that we don't recognize. Finding an anchor in God's purposes helps us establish better boundaries. "For we are His workmanship, created in Christ Jesus for good works, which God prepared beforehand so that we could walk in them." (Ephesians 2:10). The gospel narrative enables us to hear God's clear calling rather than being driven by inner forces (like professional advancement or personal ego). In the following chapters, we will explore how our identity in Christ—rather than healthcare needs and demands—can shape the direction of our work.

Bruce

Bruce grew up in a home with parents who expressed little emotion or nurturing. He became a high achiever in school. He excelled in medical school and residency, finding comfort in science's predictability and order. He preferred working on projects that did not demand emotional vulnerability. These were issues Bruce brought with him to Africa.

Bruce was a valued medical team member and eventually became the medical staff director. He was one of the few who had served long enough to appreciate the nuances of Ugandan culture. However, the desire to be culturally relevant got him into trouble; he had a bias toward Ugandan healthcare workers over expatriate workers, driven by his fear of offending Ugandans. He was not willing to hold Ugandan staff accountable for misbehavior or standards of care. His attempt to be sensitive to the culture made him afraid to challenge it.

His bias effectively generated a ministry culture that was outwardly professional but inwardly destructive. There were superior attitudes and a sense of competition, not cooperation. Rather than creating a culture of excellence, he was forming a culture of mistrust. Ministry is built on trusting relationships; experiencing trust enables us to extend trust to others. Without knowing it, Bruce was producing a toxic medical ministry culture.

When conflicts abounded, Bruce struggled to identify the source of the problem. His desire for order and predictability served him well when things were going smoothly but not in the midst of turmoil. Fear of failure kept him from connecting with others, which was essential for him as a leader. The truth was that he couldn't face emotional conflict. His own anxiety kept him from opening up to others. He wanted to give himself to love others, but it felt safer keeping more to himself.

Without healthy relationships, our blind spots often stay hidden from us. Bruce was quick to identify others' problems but not his own. He could not see how conflict avoidance and his desire for acceptance were shaping his view of reality. He would benefit from counseling in working through his personal issues as part of his own discipleship. But would he be willing to get counseling or coaching? Having achieved the status of a doctor, would he be willing to humble himself and accept help from others?

Bruce struggled to create a harmonious working culture because it demanded he dive below surface issues to the values and assumptions beneath his behavior. Here we come to the important concept of one's *worldview*, those mental maps that are almost unconscious and yet form the basis of our view of God, others, and ministry. A healthy worldview leads to healthy relationships and a healthy culture. Christians in healthcare missions with a healthy worldview must, like Christ, lead from weakness, not just from power or position.

If we allow it, *God will use conflict not to tear us down but to build us up*. You may have heard the maxim, "Use the problems to change the people rather than the people to change the problems." Embracing our own vulnerability allows God to transform us as His disciples. Our problems can change us for the better, by God's grace. The mission of healthcare is not just about providing compassionate care for those in physical need but about enabling people to become more like Jesus. We must be like Jesus first.

Learning to be like Jesus is what the Bible calls *discipleship*. It starts with evangelism (believing and receiving Jesus) and continues with a life-long process of growth in Christlikeness. Christian healthcare workers naturally want to see Jesus change the lives of patients, staff, and others in the community. But the gospel does not just change others; it changes us as well. We aren't just givers (of healthcare, gospel witness, or compassion) but we are also receivers (of healing, of grace, and of compassion).

Eventually, these changes begin to shape culture because the gospel changes culture. Obedience to Jesus Christ brings love, joy, peace, patience, and all the fruit of the Spirit. It brings holiness and righteousness. Christian values and beliefs begin to transform culture by changing hearts. (See Acts 2:43-47 for example.) Culture changes when individuals begin to work together under the leadership of the Holy Spirit; that is why Scripture emphasizes making disciples as the key command of the Great Commission.

Changing culture and behavior is not easy! The "battle" that we often experience in ministry is real. The resources are tiny compared to the need. The suffering of the people we serve is often unimaginable. The problems seem insolvable. I find it helpful to acknowledge that the work I am trying to do is impossible![7] While ministry can bring pain, it is helpful to know that Jesus uses ministry pain to shape and mold us into His image. He makes us different so that we can make a difference in others' lives.

Ultimately, this beautiful but messy call to healthcare as a ministry among the poor will lead us to a choice. Will we embrace our

---

[7] Yet with God, all things are possible. See Philippians 4:11-13

own vulnerability, brokenness, and sin? Or hide beneath position or respectability? The gospel does not leave us broken; it invites us into deeper intimacy with Jesus and more effective service to others. That's my prayer for our journey.

Yvonne

As a nursing student, Yvonne loved patient care; she loved discovering ways to share Christ, both through her words and through compassionate medical care. She began serving with this joy, assigned to work in a Nepali hospital run by a Christian non-profit. But talking to her mission leader later, she said, "I want to do community health!"

"Why? I thought you loved patient care!" he said.

"Yes, but I need to get out of the hospital!" she replied immediately.

Yvonne found herself drained by the stress of cross-cultural medicine, including conflicts among expatriates and between staff and expatriates. She wanted to escape. The joys of serving patients had faded behind clouds of uncertainty and discord.

The immediate conflicts were mostly between the expatriate and Nepali staff over resentments that had built up over the years. Paternalistic attitudes had been allowed to fester. Western values of work contrasted with local priorities about relationships; expat staff were so busy they seldom had time to build deep relationships.

Yvonne wondered if she was in the right job. She considered whether she had missed or misunderstood God's call. The emotional toll was causing her to lose focus. It was unclear to whom to bring her concerns, as most hospital leadership was already very busy.

Some fellow missionary doctors and nurses felt that "ministry" was what one did outside the hospital, in the community, or in churches. Some doctors negotiated a weekly schedule in which they spent half their time in the hospital and the other half out in the community doing "ministry." One of them made regular visits to the prison, finding fulfillment in bringing gifts and teaching the Bible to prisoners. A nurse regularly visited four villages, teaching health and encouraging local communities to identify community health volunteers she could train. Other missionary healthcare workers saw medical care as an end in itself; some saw it primarily as a means of evangelism.

It seemed like hospital and community work had little to do with each other. Yvonne felt stuck; it seemed easier to serve outside the hospital to get some relief, even though she knew little about community health. But that meant contriving her own ministry plan, as the hospital's mission was focused on the patients that arrived, not on the community.

Each healthcare worker was working with his or her own understanding of the mission purpose. Some were busy with disease care and clinical excellence. Others saw the hospital as an entry point into the community. Others stressed spiritual care. There was no common vision or purpose.

The World Health Organization (WHO) has emphasized Primary Health Care (PHC) and community health since a declaration at Alma-Ata in 1978.[8] PHC was a corrective to "the over-medicalization of health."[9] An unfortunate dichotomy was

---

[8] *Declaration of Alma-Ata.* https://www.who.int/teams/social-determinants-of-health/declaration-of-alma-ata

[9] Personal communication with Dr. Mwai Mkoka, Programme Executive for Health and Healing World Council of Churches; also see Kaczmarek E. How to distinguish medicalization from over-medicalization? Med Health Care Philos. 2019 Mar; 22(1):119-128. doi: 10.1007/s11019-018-9850-1. PMID: 29951940; PMCID: PMC6394498.

created. Ultimately, community care must go hand-in-hand with hospital or institutional care. These ministries were meant to overlap, not compete. But we will see in Chapters Nine and Ten that community health and medical care often don't share a common understanding of the mission. Without a common mission purpose, disagreement and confusion abound. A mission shaped by the story of the Bible provides the most coherent way to integrate them.

Yvonne's challenges won't be remedied by getting out of the hospital or by assuming that ministry "out there" is more spiritual than ministry "in here" in the institution. Yvonne was in a system that had not yet found how to decide what "ministry" is and how it fits into God's bigger purposes.

Finding a foundation

Do you see yourself in the stories about Cindy, Bruce, and Yvonne? Have you prioritized efficiency over joy like Cindy? Are you in need of counseling like Bruce? Are you in need of leadership because of mission drift like Yvonne?

In each story, a healthy understanding of healthcare missions is desperately needed, an understanding anchored in the bigger story of the mission of God. The bigger story provides a mental map of how the world and reality work. It helps form a healthy worldview. Theological educators Michael Goheen and Craig Bartholomew tell us, "Australian sociologist John Carroll, who does not profess to be a Christian, suggests that the reason the church in the West is in decline is because it has forgotten its story."[10]

---

[10] Goheen, M.W. and Bartholomew, C.G., *The True Story of the Whole World – Finding Your Place in the Biblical Drama* (Michigan: Brazos Press, 2020), 4.

In the following chapters, we will consider how a worldview shaped by the gospel serves as a strong foundation for healthcare missions. We will look at the gospel as a single narrative of God's ongoing redemptive work in the world. It is *this* story that gives coherence to our lives and ministry. Making this story ours is what our own discipleship is all about. Helping others learn it and make it their own is what ministry is all about. It is a unified story, a single narrative, and I hope to show how this narrative helps heal the distress we find in the lives of Bruce, Yvonne, Cindy, and even ourselves.

To close this chapter, I want to share a moving poem from Dr. David Staab, a family physician who served in Bangladesh. It speaks to the issues everyone in the healthcare mission may face at some point, issues I will address in the chapters that follow.

One More Patient
By David Staab, MD

Lord, they have asked me to see one more patient.
They really cannot take care of him themselves.
They think I have a pill for everything.
They think I know what is wrong.

The patient is a child: unwashed, underfed, unclothed, undesirable,
unneeded, uneducated, unwanted, pathetic.
He is as unwilling to be seen by me as I am unwilling to see him.
I can see the crowded boat that bore them in; a peasant's vessel,
filthy and fishy.
Tattered clothes that serve as rags for spills, and handkerchiefs
for sweat.
No need to say, "Sir, we are very poor."
This child has no diaper to catch his water that puddles on the
floor.
This family has no common sense to contain the misery that pools
up around them.

They cannot take care of him alone.
Someone has to connect them to things from far away:
Clean dry pills packaged by machines, sterile needles,
pristine fluids.
They only know of dirt and sticks and pond water.

But I have been this connection so many times before.
A well-worn bridge from poverty to technology that this patient
in a hundred different forms has crossed before.
Worn and weary, Lord, I have done and done and done.

I was comfortable.
I had done enough for a rest before this "one more" came.
My fatigue has made time a burden to me.
Even thinking is hard.

For all my Western training, my analysis is no good.
Signs and symptoms do not lead me to diagnosis and treatment.
My estimation is that this patient is hopeless and helpless.
My course of action is to remove this spectacle from my eyes.
I stand in judgment, not in Hippocratic empathy, let alone in
Christian charity.

I have no love, no compassion.
My soul is empty and not even this patient can pound on it and
get more than a dull and hollow sound, without melody or grace.

I can't.
It is a chance to spend and I am spent.
I have no hope for you, nor strength to wish you better.
Far less than a prayer to an omnipotent God that can cure, restore,
and resurrect.
Worse for you if you catch this miserable disease of heart
from me.

Lord, I am in pain.
Beyond the weariness, my heart condition speaks to me.
No hope, no love, no joy and what of peace?

The unfulfilled, selfish desires – cancer-like – consume my being.
I need… I want… I hurt from the unmet, selfish wants.
Can't you do anything for me?
Can't you? You're the Great Physician.

I am sick of heart and mind.
Unclean, ignorant, and without resources, I come to you the way this child came to me.
It's me and I am sick and I do not understand and I cannot help myself.
I need you.
I need you to see me now.
Even if you are busy.
Could you see one more patient?[11]

Questions for reflection:

What do you see in these three examples—or in this poem—that you have met in your own experience? What rings true?

What kind of struggles have you experienced in your setting? How do you feel you are coping?

---

[11] This poem originally appeared in the ABWE *Message Magazine*, Spring, 1998. Used with permission.

PART II

Discovering God's Purpose

CHAPTER 3

Created as Whole Persons, Created for Purpose

Between 2004 and 2005, I served briefly in a clinic in Thailand with an outstanding group of Thai Christian nurses, a missionary nurse, and a physician's assistant. Patients received excellent outpatient care and heard the gospel from loving workers. People were coming to Christ through the witness of the clinic. However, the mission organization that started the clinic reassigned the expatriate doctor to a different people group. Without a long-term doctor licensed in Thailand, the government shut the clinic down.

It was my privilege to help the team transition from a ministry in the clinic to one in the community. These dear servants had begun making follow-up visits to patients' homes in the surrounding hills and had established good relationships with local community leaders. The villages were Buddhist without a gospel witness; they were poor with lots of medical needs. The team continued to visit homes, met basic medical needs, and helped individuals in other ways. Some learned how to read, some learned how to play the guitar, and others learned to worship God through Bible study. The team's care for the whole person opened hearts to Christ, and many churches were planted in those hill villages.

At the start of this transition, the local church leaders raised an important question: "Why should we take time to listen and respond to the needs of the villagers?" These pastors felt that a direct gospel appeal was easier and more straightforward than all the fuss over physical needs. Why waste resources on helping people's bodies when one could just focus on evangelism and saving souls?

Those are fair questions. You may have been asked similar questions: How do medicine and the gospel fit together? If healthcare ministry is just a means to an end—introducing others to Jesus to save their souls—why not jettison healthcare when possible? Is the body that important to God? Is healthcare ministry just a way to maneuver to the "real" ministry of saving souls, or is it part of that ministry? Our search for answers will compel us to ask what God's redemptive work is all about. But before we examine God's work in redemption, we must start with God's work in creation. Creation precedes redemption, and both are part of one gospel story.

Creation is the pattern

I recently asked Dr. Bill Ardill, a surgeon who served in Nigeria for decades, to teach about integrating physical and spiritual ministry during training for healthcare missionaries. He started by turning the whole problem inside out, saying we are not trying to integrate body and soul. They have been integrated from the beginning! We were created as whole persons, whose integration begins with understanding the purpose for which we were made.

Discovering God's purpose for creation will lead us to ask about His purpose for redemption. We will find there is a unity in God's purpose that helps answer the fundamental question: What is the essence of the gospel? Working towards wholeness and integration means we must go back and understand the gospel by connecting Christ's new creation with the original.

The book of Genesis starts with God, who created one whole, integrated universe. We must start with the original design and then understand where it went wrong and how Jesus set it right. Disintegration began when humanity rebelled. The gospel is about the restoration of integration. Creation is the pattern for the *new creation* in Christ. Salvation is about restoring the creation to the purposes of God's design.

We can find ourselves perplexed because we have different expectations (or mental maps) about what God is doing to bring wholeness and integration. Theological types—pastors, church planters, and mission leaders—want to reach communities for Christ and thus stress evangelism, discipleship, and gathering groups of believers. Medical mission workers also want to see Christ worshiped but stress their own tools of the trade: patient care, health education, surgery, and medications. Ministry activities are taken from two different tool sets, with two sets of expectations.

Differing mental maps contribute to our confusion. Some healthcare ministries treat discipleship as strictly spiritual and medical care as second-rate; others value physical care so much that little time or effort goes into evangelism or building up the Body of Christ. Yet Scripture begins with both body and soul together. The creation story helps us out of our confusion by teaching us who we are as human beings and why we are here.

Who are we?

> *Then God said, "Let Us make man in Our image, according to Our likeness; and let them rule over the fish of the sea and over the birds of the sky and over the cattle and over all the earth, and over every creeping thing that creeps on the earth." God created man in his own image, in the image of God He created him; male and female He created them.*

These familiar verses from Genesis 1:26-27 reveal that God made man and woman together in His image and likeness with meaningful work to do. They were to rule wisely over creation. Humankind is to reflect God to the creation and bring creation up to the potential God intended for it.

> *Then the Lord God formed man of dust from the ground and breathed into his nostrils the breath of life, and man became a Living being [soul].* (Gen. 2:7).

Humans were created from the ground dust *and* God's breath. We are of the earth, made of the same matter as the rest of creation. But we were also created as heavenly, having received life from God. Humankind is earthly *and* heavenly – blissful integration from the start!

Rev. Dr. John W. Kleinig put it this way in his book, *Wonderfully Made: A Protestant Theology of the Body*: "We human beings are not just spirits, like the angels, nor animated bodies, like the animals, but are embodied spirits, or, if you will, spiritual bodies. We do not just have bodies; we are bodies."[12] Humankind was not created with upper and lower parts: a soul (higher, holier) and a body (unseemly, sinful). A human being is a complete person, not a body that contains a soul.[13] Kleinig continues: "The human body was made to bridge two realms: the invisible, eternal realm of God and the visible, temporal realm of creation."[14]

Psalm 8 asks, "What is man that You take thought of Him?" (v. 4). How small a human being is compared to the majesty of God. And yet, humans are uniquely appointed by God between heaven and earth. With respect to God, Psalm 8:5 states, "You have made him a little lower than God, and you crown him with glory and majesty!" With respect to creation, "You make him to rule over the works of Your hands; You have put all things under his feet, all sheep and oxen…" (Psalm 8:6-7a). Humans were made vice-regent *under* God and yet *over* creation to promote harmony between heaven and earth. Humankind has been created both as a loyal subject *and* a royal ruler. These responsibilities were aligned to enable us to display God's heaven on earth.

Theologian John Frame writes, "Thus man is designed from the beginning as perhaps the best example of integration. He is connected both to earth and heaven. He is unique in creation; no other

---

[12] John W. Kleinig, *Wonderfully Made: A Protestant Theology of the Body* (Lexham Press, 2021), 4.

[13] Soul. Not a spiritual aspect in distinction from the physical, nor the psalmist's "inner" being in distinction from his "outer" being, but his very self as a living, conscious, personal being. Its use in conjunction with "bones" (also in 35:9-10: "Soul" and "whole being") did not for the Hebrew writer involve reference to two distinct entities, but constituted for him two ways of referring to himself, as is the case also in the combination "soul" and "body" (31:9, 63:1). Barker, K. L., et al. (2002). NIV Study Bible: In *Zondervan eBooks*. https://ci.nii.ac.jp/ncid/BA7580776X

[14] Kleinig, *Wonderfully Made*, 14.

bodily creature is like him. He walks and talks with God, in person and through a gift of language which he has in common with God Himself."[15] (See Genesis 2:15-20.)

What a unique creature! Men and women are made to live under God and in a relationship with each other to accomplish God's will on earth. To be created in God's image gives great dignity to human beings, but that dignity is not ours apart from our relationship with God. We cannot find wholeness in ourselves apart from God. Our brokenness started from a broken relationship with God. That's where disintegration begins, and where we ultimately need healing. God is the "integral origin" of all things.[16] So why do humans try to separate body and soul?

Reformed philosopher and author Herman Dooyeweerd asserts that Plato's dualism—that mind and body are separate—has remained influential in the history of the Christian doctrine of creation, with the lower visible realm less 'real' than the upper, invisible one. This upper and lower hierarchy idea became *Gnosticism* – a most significant challenge to the doctrine of creation.

Years after Plato's ideas spread widely, Thomas Aquinas sought a synthesis of heaven and earthly realms but continued to split them along the lines of grace and nature. Despite Aquinas's best efforts, creation remained divided into natural and supernatural categories. The church did not fully embrace the integrated, whole understanding of humankind found in Genesis.

But it gets far worse! Five hundred years after Aquinas, Enlightenment philosophers further ruptured Aquinas's

---

[15] John M. Frame, *Systematic Theology: An Introduction to Christian Belief* (Phillipsburg: P&R Publishing, 2013), 787.

[16] Ashford, B.R. and Bartholomew, C.G., *The Doctrine of Creation* (Downers Grove: InterVarsity Press, 2020), 75.

nature-grace dualism. French mathematician and philosopher Rene Descartes formulated his theory of man as a machine.[17] In the end, philosophers discarded grace and focused on scientific reason instead of revelation from God. Truth for them was found in nature, the lower realm; science and reason became the arbiters of truth. Our understanding of reality became divided between natural (below) and supernatural (above).

In spite of all of this searching, philosophers, theologians, scientists, and everyday people were still left asking the question: Who are we? And why are we here?

Why are we here?

We have seen that the creation story is not just about how we were made (materials and mechanics) but *why* we were made. We are not defined by our bodies (like animals) but by purpose. God's purpose unifies our whole person, body and soul.

> *God blessed them; and God said to them, "Be fruitful and multiply, and fill the earth, and subdue it; and rule over the fish of the sea and over the birds of the sky and over every living thing that moves on the earth."* (Gen. 1:28).

Human beings, the pinnacle of God's creation, were not placed in God's amazing creation to live independently and do their own thing but to worship and honor God and fulfill God's purposes on earth. God had declared His creation "good," yet it was not complete. The garden was a beautiful sanctuary for man and God together,

---

[17] René Descartes *(Stanford Encyclopedia of Philosophy)*. (2023, October 23). https://plato.stanford.edu/entries/descartes/

but that beauty and communion still needed to be extended to the rest of the earth. Adam and Eve were commissioned to bring the earth to its full potential under God; their purpose was to bring the whole earth up to "garden" status. It would become a place where humankind would flourish in harmony with God's creation. God would be glorified through the flourishing of the earth. "God forms creation as a temple in which to dwell."[18]

Adam and Eve as ruling stewards were made in God's image: they were to reflect the One whose likeness they embodied. The earth is the focus and location of man's purpose, to live under God's dominion. God created us to reflect His glory on earth through a purpose directed by heaven.

Just as we would not attempt to fix equipment without understanding its function or purpose, we can only care for the whole person if we understand the role and purpose of people. Wholeness or integration is about living the life *for which God created all men and women*. We can offer meaning, not just technical skills, to others.

The physician commencement speaker at my medical school graduation in 1976 encouraged us to consider the ongoing progress of evolution and to expect progress to continue upward as medicine advances. According to his vision, science would eventually overcome human limitations and frailty. Many in the medical profession have a view of the world that puts humankind in the center of all things rather than God. True integration, however, aligns humanity's purpose with God's. "Man's chief end is to glorify God and enjoy him forever."[19]

---

[18] Ashford and Bartholomew, *The Doctrine of Creation*, 26.

[19] *Shorter Catechism with Scripture Proofs*. (2019, November). Retrieved December 4, 2023, from https://www.pcaac.org/wp-content/uploads/2019/11/ShorterCatechismwithScriptureProofs.pdf

God's glory is His brilliance, the visible evidence of His character, and the display of His goodness throughout His creation. Increasingly, we see God's glory displayed in history through the pages of the Bible. Finally, we see His glory displayed in Jesus Christ: "And the word became flesh, and dwelt among us, and we saw His glory, glory as of the only begotten from the Father, full of grace and truth." (John 1:14).

True integration aligns humanity's purpose with God's.

As Christian healthcare providers seeking to treat the whole person, we can begin to understand the nature of our task by understanding why we are here. *We are not bodies that contain souls but unique beings—body and soul together—designed to display God's glory on earth.* As providers, that means not just fixing bodies but helping others live up to their God-given purpose on earth. Let's continue to explore that purpose through what theologians call the "cultural mandate."

What is the cultural mandate?

The first missionaries to serve in Nepal in 1951 were Christian nurses. As it was a Hindu kingdom, they were allowed to meet physical needs but not to proclaim the gospel. They obeyed God's call and ministered to the poorest people with the best care they could offer. But medical care has a way of leading to conversations and trust between patient and caregiver. Before long, they could not help but share Christ's love through word as well as deed. The church there was born and began to grow; people received forgiveness, and

God's grace became known. This began to transform Nepali culture and has continued to today, over seventy years later.[20]

This is an example of the cultural mandate—we are wired for connections with others to fulfill God's will for human beings. This mandate is like a basic job description for humanity. Human beings are to work under God for the sake of human flourishing. *Human flourishing happens when men and women become whole by living under God for the sake of others and the whole creation.* This blessing is meant to go onward and outward, spreading God's goodness, justice, and righteousness throughout the world over time.

Frame says, "Man's responsibility to fill and subdue the earth is sometimes called the *cultural mandate*. That language reveals that man's task is one of turning the earth into a habitat for man, one suited to the needs and purposes of man. This task involves not only the cultivation of crops for food but also the arts, sciences, and literature, by which human life becomes more than mere subsistence. And at the deepest level, man's labor aims to bring praise and glory to God. So, he is to structure his life and culture according to God's standards."[21]

Human wholeness is more than physical wellness. It includes the intangible realities of righteousness and justice. Lovingkindness and peace are not optional afterthoughts but foundations of wholeness and flourishing. God has designed every human being—not just Christians–for this flourishing. He delights in the wellness of the body *and* the soul (remember, these are not fundamentally

---

[20] I was a missionary with the International Nepal Fellowship 1995-1997. For further stories see *Christianity in Nepal Exhibit: Yale Divinity School Library.* https://divinity-adhoc.library.yale.edu/Exhibits/Nepal_exhibit/Nepal2.htm

[21] Frame, *Systematic Theology*, 787.

separate). Wellness is not just about making individuals whole but extends to making communities and the environment whole.

When our work flows from God's creation design, we align with God as He changes people and cultures according to His purpose. God desires to bring wholeness not only to individuals but also to communities and to the natural world. We participate in the redemption of all things as we heed God's call to develop culture under His rule. "Creation is what God made out of nothing; culture is what humans make out of God's good creation."[22] Creation—this world—is still the theater of God's glory, although now pain and suffering are part of that theater too. Each of the cultures of this world is made to display the goodness of God, even in the midst of suffering. In this way, heaven and earth converge as they were designed to do.

The cultural mandate refers to our relationships as human beings with God, with one another, and with the earth. When these relationships flourish, a culture experiences *shalom*, a Hebrew word for peace. The peace of God is meant to be experienced not just personally and individually but directed outwardly to our connections with others and the environment. American theologian Cornelius Plantinga defines *shalom* as "the webbing together of God, humans, and all creation in justice, fulfillment, delight." In other words, *shalom* is "the way things ought to be."[23]

As human beings created in God's image, the cultural mandate gives shape to our call to love God and our neighbor. It should mold

---

[22] Ashford and Bartholomew, *The Doctrine of Creation*, 254.

[23] Plantinga, C., *Not the Way It's Supposed to Be: A Breviary of Sin* (Grand Rapids: Eerdmans Publishing, 1995), 10.

our special calling as medical professionals. So how does God's purpose in the creation of humankind shape our healthcare ministry?

The cultural mandate and healthcare

To start with, we can affirm the importance of the body. God cares for our bodies; they are not just containers for the soul. Ministry to the body demonstrates Jesus' compassion for those who are suffering. James describes it this way: "What use is it, my brethren, if someone says he has faith but he has no works? Can that faith save him? If a brother or sister is without clothing and in need of daily food, and one of you says to them, 'Go in peace, be warmed and be filled,' and yet you do not give them what is necessary for their body, what use is that? Even so, faith, if it has no works, is dead, being by itself."[24] Promoting health and caring for those with physical suffering combines faith and work.

Caring for bodily illness, however, requires more than technical competence. Faith expresses itself through love.[25] Loving others through illness means both caring for the body *and* believing that God is sovereignly working for His purposes in that illness. God works out His purposes through trials. We have an opportunity to help others find meaning in their suffering, as we work to grasp the patient's perspective on why he or she is ill. If we consider people as only a collection of biological and chemical elements, we reduce them to something much less than they are. We also diminish our role in working with God to help them become more fully human.

The same principle of love applies to communities. I worked with a nurse from Australia assigned to a remote government clinic

---

[24] James 2:14-17
[25] Galatians 5:6

in Ethiopia to do community health by training local health workers. She observed and advised these young men as they examined patients. It was tiresome work which she was tasked to handle alone.

She told me, "The floor is made of dirt and so uneven. As I strained for a better look at the patient, I fell off my three-legged seat."

"That was a challenge. How did you handle it?" I asked. I had been pondering how difficult it was for the rural nurses I was supervising to make a difference in the community or even in the lives of these young government health assistants.

"I don't know how many times I have fallen off that bench," she answered, without hesitation.

She took the perspective of the patient and health worker, rather than feeling sorry for herself. Her willingness to get up, dust her skirt off, and get back on that bench was a rebuke and encouragement to me. The foundation of community health is not our efforts but our love. Love means doing what God calls us to do, even when it is not glamorous.

Loving the whole person means treating him or her in relation to God, others, and the world. Care for the body cannot stop with just the body. It must extend to the purposes of God for the patient, and that brings us back to the cultural mandate. "In the Kingdom, God and His people work together to bring transformation to people and to the world."[26] We can't separate our call to care for individuals from our mandate to shape culture.

Here's an example from West Africa of how loving the whole person through healthcare might look, excerpted from a newsletter from SIM's Danja Fistula Center in Niger:

---

[26] Frame, *The Doctrine of the Christian Life*, 307.

His entire lower leg was swollen and hurting. He could not walk, so he crawled through the crowd to see the two Christian men from Danja who were visiting his village. It was immediately apparent that this 15-year-old boy had a severe lower leg and foot infection including probable bone infection. He had been suffering with this problem for months, so getting him to the hospital was the only option for treatment. He arrived at the Danja Health Center with his mother and immediately received more love, care, and attention than he had experienced in previous months. The mother commented, "Many people had seen his leg and offered no help. But when the Christians came, they showed compassion and love." She said that she had never seen love like this before and wanted to know more about becoming a Christian herself. The next day several women from this village came to visit [the boy and his mother] in the hospital. They were also amazed by the love of Christ on display and wanted to learn more about following Jesus. A few days later, the Christian men from Danja returned to the village. Previously, only the men would meet with them, but this time was different. As soon as [the Christians from Danja had] arrived in the village they were swarmed by women, all of whom had heard the testimony of the boy who'd received care in Danja. [The women, too,] wanted to hear more about the love of Jesus. This was the start of a group of women meeting in this village to learn to follow Jesus. Since then, Christian women from Danja have been able to meet with this group and help them grow in their new faith. God truly is using this health center to advance His Kingdom![27]

---

[27] Danja Health Center newsletter, May 2021, Niger, West Africa

Treating the whole person means caring for physical needs but also *speaking the truth*. It cherishes words as well as deeds. We must deeply care about suffering, both physical and spiritual. Whole-person care does not divorce material needs from deeper needs to be known, to be understood, and to be heard. It means treating each person as uniquely made in God's image, for His purpose. We get to listen to our patients' stories but also often get the opportunity to invite them to consider their suffering in the light of God's story. This means sharing meaning, purpose, and faith. Psychiatrist Viktor Frankl writes, "*Despair is suffering without meaning.*"[28] The gospel frees us from the suffering of despair.

The local church leaders I met in Thailand back in 2004 asked me, "Why should we take time to listen and respond to the needs of the villagers?" The answer is this: To enable fellow human beings to flourish under God's care is a privilege and sacred calling. This calling will bless even those who do not know God or care to follow Him. This vision is too big for any of us to do alone. Whole-person care is a group effort—from medical teams to pastors, chaplains, night nurses, and those who sweep the floor. Whether based in the hospital, the clinic, or the community, treating the whole person is ultimately designed to transform communities by God's grace and for His glory. As Christian healthcare professionals, we want to help others embrace the beauty of this calling.

Christ directs us to love others and invite them into the purpose for which they were made. Lives shaped and directed by God can change whole communities for Christ when He is lifted up. This begins to transform culture, enabling us to fulfill the cultural mandate.

---

[28] Lent, T. K. (2015). Viktor Frankl: A psychiatrist's view on how to find meaning in suffering. *Journal of Psychology & Clinical Psychiatry*. https://doi.org/10.15406/jpcpy.2015.02.00087

Questions for reflection:

Which of these themes from the chapter resonates most with you: *we are created as integrated beings; we were made to create a culture in which God is glorified and humanity flourishes; loving the whole person means treating him or her in relation to God, others, and the world; treating the whole person means caring for their physical needs and speaking the truth*? Why?

We have seen that we are created for God and others and that the cultural mandate means that we—and our patients—are created to shape the culture of the community. What difference might this make to your daily work?

CHAPTER 4

Disease, Sin, and the Corruption of Purpose

One of the assumptions I brought to my early community health efforts in Ethiopia was that programs would work. But my efforts fell flat. I've described in Chapter One how naïve expectations created much of my frustration. I was living with unhealthy beliefs about my own competence. Despite my good intentions, teaching, and good relationships, there was little change in health behaviors and no discernable change in values and attitudes underlying those behaviors. Why *does* behavior change so slowly?

It was not just that mothers withheld breast milk when children were sick or that latrines did not become plentiful, but also that many fathers remained abusive and young girls were denied education. I knew change doesn't happen easily, but it was discouraging that the community even disregarded the need for change. I expected that teaching the truth about health and the Bible–especially to the church–would have lit a fire!

But the cycle of injustice, abuse, and trauma seemed unending. Why was food not available for the kids who were malnourished? Mothers often did not know to advocate for foods that would help. Why? Because of their limited education. Why? Because they married early to get away from an abusive family situation. Why? Because the father was an alcoholic. Why? Because of an angry family feud stoked by an unjust community decision.

The pediatric ward in the hospital seemed removed from such injustice. We treated pneumonia and complications of severe malnutrition and were successful in the short range. But the "upstream" problems in the community were overpowering. We were fighting a broken and damaged system! The many wonderful things about community health I learned at the Johns Hopkins School of Public Health did not prepare me for the depth of the brokenness I would face.

As believers, we know that somehow the origins of our problems result from man's rebellion in the Garden, but that seems far removed from making a diagnosis of diabetes or screening for colorectal cancer. Why should the relationships between disease, suffering, and sin make a difference to us as healthcare professionals?

What is sin?

In the last chapter, we considered how God made us whole persons, body and soul, to fulfill His purpose on earth, creating a culture in which God is glorified and humanity flourishes. Adam and Eve's rebellion, however, set them on a pathway of death and separation from God and His purpose for them.

> *The serpent said to the woman, "You surely will not die! For God knows that in the day you eat from it your eyes will be opened and you will be like God, knowing good and evil."* (Gen. 3:4-5).

The "Fall" of Adam and Eve recorded in Genesis 3 recounts their choice to "be like God" in their own way rather than God's. Like Satan, they chose to trust themselves, disobeying God's command. They fell from their integrated relationship and communion with God through this sin. Separated from His life-giving presence, they were banished to a pathway leading to death–not just physical death but the death of their entire personhood, body and soul. This distorted their relationships with each other and creation. Their action cast all of humanity into a life-long struggle with sin (i.e., to maintain control without God).

In trying to be like God on their own terms, they corrupted the human race, whom God cast out from the Garden as a consequence of the Fall. Human beings began to experience shame and separation, pain in childbirth, thorns, and thistles, bread made by the sweat of their brow, and physical death. Their sin was a "whole-person" event, corrupting us as humans and making it impossible for us to flourish by ourselves. Salvation would need to address the whole person to bring us back into alignment with the purposes of God. Thankfully, the same good God that specified the consequences also promised deliverance from sin and Satan through the seed of the woman.[29]

The German theologian Erich Sauer explained life after the Fall in this way: "There follows, with the entrance of the Fall, a

---

[29] Genesis 3:15

'fixed association between spiritual and bodily distress, between inward and outward injury, between world-guilt and world-sorrow, between human sin and groaning creation.'"[30] Or, as Frame says succinctly, "This cosmic disruption is an index of the seriousness of sin."[31]

Without the Fall, we would have no work as healthcare providers, since disease is coupled with death. And yet, without God's promise of salvation, we would have no hope. Our quest as Christian healthcare workers is to work in hope, helping those suffering from the effects of the Fall connect with the reality of grace.

In his book *Are Christians Human?*, Nigel M. de S. Cameron tells us that Adam was already, "as like God as ever a creature could be."[32] Human beings could not rise higher than the station that God appointed them. "There is no higher station open to any creature."[33]

Sin does not change our essential nature or make us "unhuman." We are still in the image of God, although that image is now distorted or corrupted. Biblical scholars Ashford and Bartholomew remind us that "sin does not have the power to make bad what God has made good. It can only misdirect God's creation toward bad ends."[34] Sin does not change the purpose for which God made us; it corrupts it. Despite the Fall, God still calls us to rule and fulfill the cultural mandate to make the earth flourish.

---

[30] Sauer, Erich., *The Dawn of World Redemption: A Survey of the History of Salvation in the Old Testament* (Grand Rapids: Eerdmans Publishing, 1951), 57.

[31] Frame, *Systematic Theology*, 859.

[32] Nigel M. de S. Cameron, *Are Christians Human?* (Grand Rapids: Zondervan Publishing, 1988), 111.

[33] Ibid., 111.

[34] Ashford, *Doctrine of Creation*, 231.

Plantinga helps us see the effects of sin, not just personally but between people: "God hates sin not just because it violates his law, but, more substantively, because it violates *shalom*, because it breaks the peace, because it interferes with the way things are supposed to be... God is for *shalom* and *therefore* against sin. In fact, we may safely describe evil as any spoiling of *shalom*, whether physically (e.g., by disease), morally, spiritually, or otherwise... *In short, sin is culpable shalom-breaking.*"[35]

> **Our quest as Christian healthcare workers is to work in hope, helping those suffering from the effects of the Fall connect with the reality of grace.**

Sin does not manifest itself only in our soul, as if it were possible to separate soul and body. Neither does it manifest only by the disease and death of the body. Sin pervades the whole person; it is our most persistent enemy. It is "the longest-running of all human emergencies."[36] Furthermore, sin is not just about my personhood but affects all human relationships, even causing the creation to groan. An ecology of sin shows that we are vulnerable to Satan and his celestial rebellion, fostering his destructive purposes for humanity.[37]

Consider sexual abuse. Sin (abusive behavior) is rebellion against God's creation since it defaces one of God's precious creatures. But that abuse causes a cascade of other effects, which can

---

[35] Plantinga, *Not the Way It's Supposed to Be: A Breviary of Sin*, 14. [Italics mine]
[36] Ibid., 5.
[37] O'Neill, D.W. "Sin and the Etiology of Disease" in *All Creation Groans: Toward a Theology of Disease and Global Health*, O'Neill, D.W. and Snodderly, B., eds. (Eugene: Pickwick Publications, 2021).

lead to mental, physical, social, and relational dysfunction or disease. Suffering and illness are connected back to sin through a complex web of intermediate causes.

Sin and its corruption are the roots of disordered behavior and culture. Moral evil becomes the root of all sorts of natural and physical evil. Thorns and thistles are not sins in themselves but are the effects of sin and remind us of the pain of our separation from God. Breast cancer is not sin itself but is connected to sin through a cascade of intermediate brokenness. The brokenness may be morally evil (such as abuse) or morally neutral (such as DNA mutations). There are often layers of brokenness between sin and disease, much of which we barely understand.

This means that diagnosing diabetes or screening colorectal cancer really isn't *that* far removed from humanity's rebellion against God.

What is disease?

The Oxford English dictionary defines disease as "disturbance or impairment of the function (and often also the structure) of the body, a part of the body, or the mind."[38] We make sense of the world by recognizing natural causes, rooted in the body's biology, chemistry, and physiology. DNA gets broken, causing mutations. COVID variants develop into new pandemic waves. Lead in pipes damages brains and limits human capacity. These material causes of disease, however, are often rooted in deeper causes that are real but may not be material.

---

[38] *Disease*, Oxford English Dictionary, www.oed.com/dictionary/disease_n#eid (2023, July).

Disease can have roots in the mind, emotions, or relationships. In the late 1990s, before the advent of antiretrovirals, I helped SIM develop a multi-country approach to HIV and AIDS called "HOPE for AIDS." We described the problem as a disease of broken relationships. The brokenness we experience as human beings is not just physical but also personal. We are broken people, not broken machines.

The brokenness underlying our diseases may ultimately be the result of human sin, but the diseases are not sin itself. Disease is an expression of natural evil or brokenness. Natural evil is connected to moral evil (sin) but the two are not the same. The scourge of HIV and AIDS is not a sin but rather an expression of disorder in our persons, which is ultimately an expression of humanity's rebellion. The same goes for neonatal tetanus, osteoarthritis, or any of a thousand expressions of our human frailty.

As Christians, we must bring wisdom, not just science, to the bedside. When the Ebola epidemic raged in Liberia in 2014, communities continued to be infected by their death ritual of washing the bodies of the dead. They were more fearful of abandoning traditional practices than Ebola. The cause of the epidemic on one level was the ongoing viral transmission. On another level, it was the cultural practices and beliefs about honoring the dead. SIM missionaries and Liberian staff treated many patients successfully, but medical care alone could not have stopped the outbreak. The tide began to turn only when local volunteers, along with local pastors, helped communities modify their practices to *both* honor their dead and respect the epidemiology of the disease. Scientific logic without social and cultural explanations would not have worked.[39]

Our privilege as Christian healthcare providers is to treat the whole person. Physical symptoms can become a door through which we address non-physical causes. Family dysfunction often distorts healthy human relationships later in life. Systemic racial injustice tears at the image of God in human beings in many ways. Greed and abuse of power frequently deflect health resources from those who need them most. While we cannot be specialists for every trauma and injustice, we may be able to empower the patient and others to tackle root issues. Theologian Henri Nouwen says, "Perhaps the main task of the minister is to prevent people from suffering for the wrong reasons."[40]

A Christian view of disease and illness recognizes the complexity of multiple causes—not just biological causes, not just sinful causes, but a matrix of factors. Consider Jesus' response to the disciples' question about who was to blame that the man was born blind. He answered, "It was neither that this man sinned, nor his parents; but it was so that the works of God might be displayed in him."[41] Jesus did not deny that there were physical causes of the man's blindness; neither did He interpret his blindness as only spiritual in nature. He likely recognized multiple dimensions of his blindness, including human sin. But He lifted the conversation beyond either-or causes to focus His healing on the glory of God.

---

[39] I served on the SIM US Ebola emergency response team. Also see: Jansen, P. "The Role of Faith-Based Organizations and Faith Leaders in the 2014-2016 Ebola Epidemic in Liberia". Christian Journal for Global Health, vol. 6, no. 1, May 2019, pp. 70-78, https://doi.org/10.15566/cjgh.v6i1.265

[40] Nouwen, Henri J.M., *The Wounded Healer* (Garden City: Image Books, 1979), 93.

[41] John 9:3

British pastor and physician Dr. Martyn Lloyd-Jones describes the roots of disease and suffering like this: "Man's real problem is not simply that he is sick, but that he is a rebel. Now here again is a crucial distinction. The current notion is that humanity is sick. And of course, it is sick, very sick indeed. The real question, however, is why is it sick? The basic answer of the Bible and the church, when she is really preaching the Bible, is that man's ultimate problem is not sickness. That is only a symptom or a complex of symptoms. It is a manifestation of something much deeper and more serious."[42]

Sin and disease are often connected through a variety of intermediary causes. Some of these causes are sinful and others are just brokenness because of our human condition. Let's consider these connections first on an individual patient level and then on a community level.

Connecting disease and sin in the patient

A modern approach to medical care focuses on material mechanisms and cannot answer life's ultimate questions, such as, "Who am I? Why am I here? Why do I suffer?" because it is reductionistic. Life is compartmentalized, and such questions are either left unanswered or the patient is left to think that his or her illness is from random chance. We have the honor of addressing these questions as we care for the suffering. We are not responsible for providing final answers to questions that cannot be answered. God has a way of communicating His sovereignty and goodness even during pain like He did for Job in the Old Testament.

---

[42] Martin Lloyd-Jones, *Healing and the Scriptures* (Nashville: Thomas Nelson, 1988), 64.

But what about communities that do not see life as compartmentalized between the sacred and secular? We often serve in cultures around the globe that see life more as a unified whole. What do we need to understand about these cultures? How might they understand illness?

Animistic worldviews dominate many cultures worldwide, sometimes under a veneer of a major religion such as Islam, Hinduism, and even sometimes Christianity. Animistic people attribute the cause of illness to spirits or curses. They attempt to manipulate the spirit world out of fear, through charms, amulets, and magic. Among the Bunna tribe in remote southern Ethiopia, neonatal tetanus was common. It was thought that the umbilicus after birth was a route for evil spirits to enter the baby, and so dirt was applied to the fresh umbilical stump from under the doorway of the house. They reasoned that the spirits that control the house entrance could also be relied on to control malicious spirits entering the baby. (For those who are not medically trained, the soil is the source of tetanus bacilli.) What an amazing opportunity to announce the good news of the gospel! We can affirm the reality of the spirit world and show how through death, Jesus has risen victorious over the leader of that world. The gospel has provided salvation to many Bunna people as well as practical deliverance from the fear of evil spirits. Disease and death are not outside the sovereign purposes of a good God.

Shame-based cultures frequently view illness directly as a result of personal sin. Indian karma may attribute the death of a young man in a car crash to his previous sins. This perspective distracts from important causes, such as road safety, lack of seat belts, or texting while driving. While we can't be dogmatic, a sensitive Christian can receive the family's pain and explore their beliefs and misgivings, often opening an opportunity to speak words from God. I have seen families begin to soften to the message of God's grace through such tragedies. How we interpret illness matters.

Professor and orthodox Christian Jean-Claude Larchet takes the discussion further: "Every form of illness causes suffering. Most cause us to suffer both physically and psychologically. All of them create spiritual suffering since they reveal, sometimes with a certain cruelty, the fragile nature of our condition. They remind us that health and biological life are not 'goods' that we can hold on to forever, but that in this world our body is destined to diminish, to deteriorate, and finally to die."[43] Illness is a theater that needs proper interpretation! Suffering and illness force us to ask the question "why?" "What is the meaning or purpose of my illness?"

It is as Larchet said, "By virtue of illness, man comes back to himself."[44] Illness and suffering invite us to consider a complex web of causes. Not all of these causes will be connected to personal sin, although all of them will eventually be traceable back to the Fall. This web of brokenness can provide a window into our patient's life and may suggest ways to communicate the narrative of God's work in the world. While we cannot answer all questions, our love can help others find hope in God's providential hand working through the illness toward His good purpose. Ultimately death, the final enemy, has been defeated because sin has been put away at the cross.

---

[43] Jean-Claude Larchet, *The Theology of Illness* (St Vladimir's Seminary Press, 2002), 9.

[44] Ibid., 52.

Connecting disease, sin, and community

Sin is not just an individual, personal reality but a corporate one. Humanity itself is lost in sin, leading to broken communities. Sin disrupts *shalom*. By nature, we are *shalom*-breakers; thus, without Christ, human beings make cultures that destroy life rather than give it. The disruption of *shalom* demonstrates the awful reality of our rebellion against God and calls believers to be salt and light in the world.

Reformed philosopher Herman Dooyeweerd describes this loss of universal flourishing. "Sin corrupts progressively, not limiting itself to the private self but extending to the public self and ultimately to society and culture. It is like cancer in that it is a dynamic and relentlessly progressive phenomenon that reproduces rapidly and leaves the aroma of death in its wake."[45] How shortsighted we are if we treat the symptoms of a cancer but not the cancer itself!

If you have spent time in healthcare missions, you've likely seen the corruption of sin in public life already. Many of the diseases we encounter have root causes in the disruption of *shalom*.

This is even true for tuberculosis, a disease caused by one bacterium. A growing consensus is that tuberculosis control requires effective drug treatment *and* attention to issues such as poverty, crowding, and population mobility. We refer to these roots as the *social determinants* of disease. Poverty, lack of education, abuse, injustice, greed, and ethnic hatred are just a few of these. Practical ideas for action can't be found simply by treating the biology of tuberculosis, but by addressing these other underlying causes. Human flourishing can be advanced by community treatment of

---

[45] Ashford, *Doctrine of Creation*, 237.

tuberculosis, advocating for better housing, or fighting the injustices behind urban crowding. Each of these approaches allows us to connect our activities with the narrative of God's *shalom*, sin, and redemption. Our vision is to make disciples who care about these things as well. We want to lead efforts to pray for and support those who are working for *shalom* in the community. Ultimately, God changes culture towards *shalom* through many disciples of Christ working together.

Why is this important?

Connecting disease and sin–and having the tools to do so–can make a big difference in how we practice. For starters, it provides a framework for us to understand disease *both* as a biological *and* a relational happening. It keeps us from making the mistake of equating disease with sin yet encourages us to identify and address sin when we find it at the root. It gives us a way of bringing the whole person together as dignified and made in the image of God and yet as broken and in need of the healing that Jesus provides. It gives us language to address suffering and pain at a deeper level.

While disease focuses on biological mechanisms, illness is a broader term. Illness "refers to how the sick person and the family or wider social network members perceive, label, experience, and respond to symptoms and disability…Disease and illness can express different interpretations of a single clinical reality…"[46] In treating people, we can help them interpret *both* their disease *and* their illness. Pain, for example, can be a physiological symptom, but it also carries meaning for the person. Treating the whole person

---

[46] Rhee, H., *Illness, Pain and Health Care in Early Christianity* (Grand Rapids: Eerdmans Publishing, 2022), 5.

means addressing not just biological roots but the meaning of the pain to the individual. We should do our best to treat the person from both perspectives. As C.S. Lewis said, "God whispers to us in our pleasures, speaks in our conscience, but shouts in our pains: it is His megaphone to rouse a deaf world."[47]

In 1946, Dr. Nathan Barlow reopened a medical work in Soddo, southern Ethiopia, which Italian forces had shut down during World War II. Soon after he arrived, Barlow saw the needs in the communities beyond the hospital. After prayer and discussions with the local (SIM-related) Word of Life Church leaders, he began discussions with the Ethiopian Ministry of Health about opening a training center for rural health workers. Permission was granted for a two-year training and discipleship program. Many of the graduates were Christians and were assigned to operate clinics back in their respective districts. The local population received help with malaria, TB, dysentery, typhus, and other common diseases. Severe cases were referred to the Soddo Hospital. These rural health assistants made a significant contribution to the work of the gospel in southern Ethiopia through the care they gave for both body and soul. Many of them became trusted leaders in local churches.[48]

These leaders modeled Jesus: He cares not only about physical illness but also about the person who is sick. Illness becomes a megaphone through which God speaks to us. God puts the call to repentance into a language everyone understands—the language of

---

[47] Lewis, C.S., *The Problem of Pain* (Harper Collins UK, 1998).

[48] This is a story I told in Chapter 19, "Ministries of Compassion" in *By Prayer to the Nations*, Gary R. Corwin, ed. (Grand Rapids: Credo Publishers, 2018), 274-299.

pain and death.[49] He genuinely cared for the legs of the paralyzed man whose friends let him down on a pallet through the roof in Mark 2. But he also cared for the man's deeper need—forgiveness from sin. He healed him not only to show that he cared about his diseased body but also to confirm his friends' faith and challenge his enemies' unbelief. He treats the whole person, not just the body or soul separately.

As followers of Christ, we can grow to be best at treating the whole person, helping him or her hear God's voice. We can learn to treat others with dignity as created in God's image and yet with patience as sinners. In his Doctor's Casebook, Swiss physician and influential Christian author Paul Tournier said that "technical treatment and human sympathy are not enough. The mission of the doctor is wider still. Helping a person to live does not mean only helping him to bear his life, but helping him to grow and to solve his problems."[50]

Dr. Mark Topazian teaches gastroenterology and disciples students and residents in Addis Ababa, Ethiopia. He told me that Christian medical students in Ethiopia are eager to serve the Lord, but some don't understand how to do so in the hospital.

I asked him, "Why would they not consider work in the hospital as a ministry?" I had assumed that, like me, they might not see much connection between sin and disease. I was surprised by Mark's answer.

---

[49] John Piper is riffing off Lewis's well-known turn of phrase that pain is God's megaphone. Piper J., *Providence* (Wheaton: Crossway Books, 2020), 504.

[50] Paul Tournier, *A Doctor's Casebook in Light of the Bible* (Harper and Row, Publishers, 1954), 181.

Mark said, "Many Christian medical students *do* think that disease and sin are connected–in fact, some tend to think that patients are in the hospital because God is punishing them."

"So, they see God's hand in disease but don't see it as an invitation to connect with patients on a deeper level," I mused.

Mark responded, "It's more a matter of what constitutes healing. Many see that medicine by itself is not enough. They believe that real, complete healing requires repentance and happens in a church. Within the constraints of a secular healthcare institution, Christian students here don't have the tools they need to learn about and encourage their patients' spiritual health in a contextually acceptable fashion. It's my job to equip them for that."[51]

Now, all this talk of treating the whole person and talking about the meaning of illness may be unsettling. You may ask, "How can I possibly do more than my busy schedule allows? It only makes the burden greater. How can this be an encouragement?" I hope that by changing your perspective on treating patients, you will connect with patients and staff in deeper ways and find more satisfaction in your work. Aligning with God's purposes for ministry does not mean doing more work but rather connecting more deeply with the people God has already given us. It is an invitation to deepen relationships with God and others.

Human effort alone cannot bring *shalom* without addressing brokenness and sin. To our modern ears, it may sound judgmental to call attention to sin, but we must face it squarely if we are to be Kingdom disciples. Jesus did not hesitate to talk about sin, hell, or judgment. If we avoid these topics, we miss the opportunity to bring God's solution to the root causes of disease–sin and

---

[51] Dr. Mark Topazian, personal communication, Oct 5, 2022

corruption. The gospel is the power of God for salvation from sin and for *shalom*.

Whether we are doctors or hospital volunteers, whether we work with shiny new technology or flip charts, we can find ways to communicate the gospel better by connecting with others in their brokenness. The gospel is the power to change people and communities. Disciples eventually transform cultures. Whatever we are doing, we have a small part in a broad work of redemption, moving culture and history in real-time according to God's purposes.

As we continue to examine healthcare ministry through the lens of the gospel, we will discover that ministry is a community or team effort, not just our own. Dr. Barlow was able to look at the real needs of the patients and see the deeper needs of the community–both for physical health and for salvation from sin. God used Dr. Barlow's relationship with other believers in Soddo, Ethiopia, to work for lasting change in the region for God and for good. God can use us this way, too.

Questions for reflection:

Sin does not just corrupt the body but our whole purpose as human beings. How might caring for others allow us to connect them with that purpose?

Illness becomes a megaphone through which God speaks to us. What might you do this week to help someone hear God speaking?

CHAPTER 5

Health, Salvation, and Restoration of God's Purpose

Healing is not just confined to the physical domain; it invites us to see God at work and give Him glory. It can be interpreted either with spiritual sight or spiritual blindness. Jesus healed a blind man, who then told his neighbors: "The man who is called Jesus made clay, and anointed my eyes, and said to me, 'Go to Siloam and wash'; so I went away and washed, and I received my sight."[52] These facts about his healing were not in dispute. It was the interpretation of the facts that was controversial. The objective facts were met with either faith or unbelief.

The Jewish leaders verified the man's physical healing by speaking to him and his parents but refused to attribute the healing to

---

[52] John 9:11

Jesus. They said to the man, "You are his disciple, but we are disciples of Moses."[53]

Jesus used the healing miracle to open the spiritual eyes of the blind man and to reveal His goodness and love. He said to him, "Do you believe in the Son of Man?" The man answered, "Who is He, Lord, that I may believe in Him?"[54] Choosing belief over doubt, the man found salvation and forgiveness of sin. Yet, Jesus warned the Pharisees, "Since you say 'We see,' your sin remains."

My anatomy, physiology, and pathology training make it natural for me to attribute healing strictly to biological forces. Early intervention in typhoid fever prevents intestinal perforation. Penicillin makes gram-positive bacteria fragile and more easily defeated by the immune system. How does the healing I witness as a medical professional speak about spiritual sight and salvation? How do I interpret healing with spiritual eyes?

What is healing?

You are likely familiar with WHO's definition of health as "a state of complete physical, mental and social well-being and not merely the absence of disease or or infirmity."[55] This definition addresses human well-being in multiple dimensions, although it leaves out the spiritual dimension. Healing must address not just human well-being but God's purpose for our well-being. Healing restores our bodies to the way things are supposed to function, designed for us to serve God and others. Healing reminds us of the way things are supposed to be, prompting us to consider God's

---

[53] John 9:28

[54] See John 9:35-38

[55] WHO Constitution, 1948

original design and purpose for us and show how we have fallen short of that design. It helps us look forward as well as backward. Healing points us to the future when God will restore all things in a new creation in Christ.

> *Healing is the restoration of body, mind, or spirit to a state of wholeness and well-being. This restoration may be physical, as in the recovery from an illness or injury, or spiritual, as in the forgiveness of sins and justification before God. Ultimately, healing is embodied by Jesus, as He healed the sicknesses of many in His earthly ministry and secured ultimate healing for all in His death on the cross and subsequent resurrection.*[56]

I find it astounding that God created our bodies to heal. Even when we give antibiotics, the natural immune system must be activated to clean up the infection. The surgeon makes the cut, but God has made the body so that the edges grow back together. As Nepal's Tansen Hospital proclaims, "We treat, Jesus heals." Healing speaks to us much more about God than it does about the doctors and nurses He may use to bring healing.

Healing puts us in the middle of the story of God's work from creation to the new creation. Healing goes beyond making the right diagnosis or therapy. It has meaning because it is a gift from God to restore us to life and His purposes. Thus, it calls for our gratitude.

Adam and Eve's spiritual death—their separation from God—followed immediately from their sin, but physical death was delayed. God in His grace did not wipe them out immediately.

---

[56] C. Byrley, "Healing" in D. Mangum, D. R. Brown, R. Klippenstein, & R. Hurst (Eds.), *Lexham Theological Wordbook* (Bellingham: Lexham Press, 2014).

Adam lived over 930 years,[57] and perhaps Eve's lifespan was similar. God gave them time to live, have children, till the ground, and begin to make a culture so that the earth would flourish. But sin was like an anchor dragging the boat backward. Childbirth would be painful. Agriculture would be exhausting. Thorns and thistles would thwart them. They likely would have needed healing many times during their lives.

Adam and Eve's life was not an inexorable downward path to death. God built the possibility of healing into their bodies at creation. Although we may often take it for granted, God designed our bodies to recover from illness. Consider macrophages, for instance. These immune cells live on standby for tissue injury and repair.[58] We are just beginning to appreciate the complex ways they communicate with other cells and each other.

Healing for Adam and Eve enabled them to live for God, not just for themselves. God worked in their lives to restore them to Himself and to enable them to reflect His glory in the world. They would not have been able to serve God without receiving healing from illness and accident. Neither could they obey Him without forgiveness of sin. Healing and salvation both restore life and purpose to the human race. Together, they are components of God's singular design.

Healing is not a right but a gift. It is not simply an outcome of our efforts but rather a work of God. It is not a hard-wired program in the human body; it's an ongoing message to us from heaven.

---

[57] Genesis 5:5

[58] Watanabe S, Alexander M, Misharin AV, Budinger GRS. *The role of macrophages in the resolution of inflammation.* J Clin Invest. 2019 May 20;129(7):2619-2628. doi: 10.1172/JCI124615. PMID: 31107246; PMCID: PMC6597225.

What is salvation?

Salvation is whole-person healing. The Old Testament uses the Hebrew word for salvation as deliverance from military victory or danger in general. The New Testament word for salvation means not only health, safety, and deliverance from danger but also deliverance from the penalty and power of sin. In both Testaments, salvation is holistic and involves the whole person's well-being, not just his mind or spirit.[59]

When Jesus healed the woman with the hemorrhage of twelve years, "immediately the flow of blood was dried up; and she felt in her body that she was healed of her affliction."[60] Jesus healed more than her physical affliction. She came to Him trembling with fear and shame. "He said to her, 'Daughter, your faith has made you well; go in peace [*eirene*] and be healed of your affliction.'"[61] He called her "daughter," taking away not only her sickness but her shame. He gave her worth and restored her to God as well as to society. This was whole-person medicine at its best!

Praise God that salvation is spiritual. It must be since it comes from heaven and directs us to God. Without Christ's sacrifice on the cross, we would be eternally lost. But as modern people, we tend to think that salvation is *only* spiritual, something that happens to the soul but has no real effect on the body or the material world. But Nigel Cameron reminds us, "The purpose of redemption is to

---

[59] Hamme, J.T., "Salvation" in D. Mangum, D. R. Brown, R. Klippenstein, & R. Hurst (Eds.), *Lexham Theological Wordbook* (Bellingham: Lexham Press, 2014).

[60] Mark 5:29

[61] Mark 5:34

enable man to be once more himself, restored to his right mind and his right place as a creature of God."[62]

We sometimes make salvation a private transaction that occurs between us and God, having little to do with how we live our lives in the body. This is not what Jesus preached as the good news of the Kingdom. The good news is that Jesus has won the victory over death and has been coronated as King! His Kingdom is not just a spiritual, invisible one. It changes people as a whole—body and soul—and orients them toward God's purpose in this world and the next.

> **Healing is an ongoing message to us from heaven.**

Jonathan Edwards helps us better understand salvation (or redemption) by describing it in two ways. Salvation can be viewed narrowly in terms of Christ's finished work on the cross. It can also be viewed more broadly as the work of God over the course of history. Both views of salvation are founded on Christ and flow from His cross. The narrower view focuses us on what God has done to accomplish this great work. The broader view helps us tie salvation with God's objective work in history; He restores human beings and creation from the ruins of the Fall. God's design connects the salvation of sinners and the building of His Kingdom.[63]

Let's look at an example that ties salvation in with the broader work of God in history. Social scientist Robert Woodbury has done extensive research on the historical roots of democracy, challenging other theories. Traditional theories of democracy stress "the

---

[62] De S. Cameron, *Are Christians Human?*, 110.

[63] Jonathan Edwards, *A History of the Work of Redemption*. (Hardpress Publishing, 2013), 11-26.

importance of secular rationality, economic development, urbanization, industrialization and the expansion of the state."[64] He provides solid evidence that while these factors may be important, Western modernity itself is shaped by religious factors, especially Protestant missionary activity whose purpose was religious conversion. His research "demonstrates historically and statistically that Conversionary Protestants (CPs) heavily influenced the rise and spread of stable democracy around the world. It argues that CPs were a crucial catalyst, initiating the development and spread of religious liberty, mass education, mass printing, newspapers, voluntary organizations, and colonial reforms, thereby creating the conditions that made stable democracy more likely."[65] Salvation does not just affect individuals but cultures.

Salvation is not just personal restoration to God but the restoration of creation. God is making a new creation in place of the original fallen creation. He will not just restore creation to the original model; God's new creation will enhance the original garden design in ways we cannot yet fathom. Because Jesus has risen from the dead, the victory over sin has been won. In His time, the earth will know the blessings of heaven. When Christ returns, he will fully restore and transform the earth.

Neither separate nor identical

Healing and salvation are neither separate nor identical. Each looks at the whole person from a different perspective. As healthcare

---

[64] Woodbury, R.D. The Missionary Roots of Liberal Democracy. American Political Science Review, Vol 106, No 2, May 2012, p. 244. See DOI: https://doi.org/10.1017/S0003055412000093

[65] Ibid., 244.

workers, we grasp that healing and salvation are closely related, and it helps to know they are part of God's one story. But we also need to distinguish them carefully.

Plantinga puts it so well: "Sin makes us guilty while disease makes us miserable."[66] Sickness is depressing but it is not sin. As we have seen in an earlier chapter, sickness is a result of human brokenness, but sin is the ultimate cause of that brokenness.

All people die. Healing of the body is always temporary until that final day when we return, like Adam, to dust. Although it is temporary, healing points us to our need, our frailty, and our dependence on God. Healing is not permanent until believers receive resurrection bodies from God; salvation points us to that future hope.

In a sense, healing is always partial. Even when we are well, our bodies are still in the process of dying. Lazarus, whom Christ raised from the dead, died again later. Salvation is not partial; it is complete and lasts eternally. Raising Lazarus from the dead was truly miraculous but only foreshadowed the greater miracle of Jesus' own death and resurrection. Lazarus' healing also foreshadows his eventual resurrection when Jesus returns.

Healing makes us hopeful but doesn't remove sin. Salvation anchors our hope because it addresses sin at the root level.

Bodily healing is more tangible and obvious to us; pain gets our attention more readily than our spiritual needs. Salvation is the deeper but often the less obvious need.

Healing and salvation are not automatically linked. Our efforts to heal may fail (since a cure is not always possible and death is never that far away). But salvation is assured since it is based on

---

[66] Plantinga, *Not the Way It's Supposed to Be*, 20.

Jesus' finished work on the cross. God does not always heal our bodies upon request, but He never fails to answer us when we call on Him for salvation. We can be saved without being physically healed. We can experience God's *shalom* in the midst of bodily brokenness and intractable illness.

My mother was saved but died of Alzheimer's disease. Yet in her dementia, she had child-like joy and a good relationship with my father. From that perspective, she was fully "healed" before being with the Lord.

Jesus healed ten lepers, but only one turned back to give thanks. Jesus said, "Were there not ten cleansed? But the nine–where are they? Was no one found who returned to give glory to God, except this foreigner?"[67] Through healing, Jesus was inviting them to turn to Him for salvation. While the nine received healing, they did not receive salvation. Their bodies were restored but the direction of their lives away from God did not change.

Healing leads us to a bigger salvation story

High on a Tibetan plateau, I was part of a small group of medical missionary doctors and nurses invited to treat ill villagers. We were hampered by a lack of lab tests and limited diagnostic equipment. We had carried some select antibiotics and acetaminophen up the mountainside but not enough to meet the need. I remember vividly a young woman in her twenties with crippling rheumatoid arthritis. No medical care was available; we had to make do with giving her aspirin. After taking a history (through translation) and

---

[67] Luke 17:17-18

making our diagnoses, we were allowed to pray for her and many other patients in the name of Jesus.

Several weeks later, after we returned to the city, we were given some follow-up on the village. It was amazing how many had recovered; some had completely healed! This young woman experienced total remission. God's miracle!

I understood how much God cared for those I considered lost or forgotten. Though they were not rich by the world's standards and were enslaved to the spirits they worshiped, God loved them and wanted their salvation. He spoke to them through our simple words and deeds.

As we have seen, bodily healing and salvation both flow from God's gracious plan to restore human beings to Himself and enable them to glorify God on earth. Both aim to restore human wholeness or integrity, broken by the Fall. Both are made possible by Jesus because of His sacrifice on the cross. Both flow from God's love.

Yet, while bodily healing is part of the story, it is not the end of the story—hallelujah! It is not the final story. It is a megaphone through which God speaks to us of a promise found only in Christ. It becomes part of a narrative that speaks of hope and invites us to trust Him as the only one who makes people truly whole. It speaks of God's glorious future and also His present glories.

The future of our salvation story is free from suffering and death. This earth (with its corruption) will pass away, sin and evil will be purged away, and everything redeemable renewed and transformed at Christ's appearing. The Apostle John describes the new heaven and the new earth in Revelation 21 after this restoration: "He will wipe away every tear from their eyes; and there will no longer be any death; there will no longer be any mourning, or crying, or pain; the first things have passed away."[68]

It is not just our patients that need this good news but we ourselves. As healthcare professionals, we can lose the story and lose our way. A vital connection with Jesus will encourage us day by day, even when there are not enough workers and malaria season threatens to overrun us.

The same salvation story is not only about the future but also about the present. The Kingdom of God is coming, but it is also at hand. God is preparing individuals for heaven (Hallelujah!) and preparing a people to show His glory on earth now. The story is not just about what Jesus has done for me but what He is doing to renew creation now. Since His glory will cover the earth—*this earth*—in the future, salvation today is a preview of that final day. Healing today reveals something of the character of the coming Kingdom of God.

After you received salvation, maybe you wondered, like me, why God did not bring you directly to heaven. This is the answer: The gospel of the Kingdom doesn't remove us *from* the world but enables us to live for Christ *in* this world. As His disciples, we pray, "Thy Kingdom come, Thy will be done on earth as it is in heaven." Our part is to offer the needy a cup of cold water and tell them where to find living water (see John 4:14).

The Kingdom of God is where "God supernaturally carries through His supremacy against all opposing powers and brings man to the willing recognition of the same. It is the state of things

---

[68] Revelation 21:4

in which everything tends towards God as the greatest good."[69] *The Kingdom of God is not what we can do for God—even through the marvels of modern medicine—but what God carries out on the earth through us, the Body of Christ.* The focus is not on our works and ability but on God's. "Man was put on the earth to make a name for God, not for himself."[70]

The Great Commission (to make disciples who obey Jesus) and the Great Commandment (to love our neighbor) are part of a single story. We love others by enabling them (through God's grace at work in us) to flourish; this is God's design for humanity from creation. The purpose is to create a world that thrives under God. The Great Commission enables us to fulfill the creation (cultural) mandate by getting to the heart of our trouble: sin.

God uses the result of sin (disease, suffering, and death) to defeat sin itself by pointing the world to its need for a Savior. And the disciples of the Savior obey Him and are enabled, by grace, to help the world to flourish. This one story starts from creation and moves to the restoration of that creation in Christ. That restoration began at the cross and will ultimately be completed when Jesus returns to earth in glory.

Jesus describes the character of the Kingdom of God in the Sermon on the Mount. This paints a picture of God's design for the people and cultures of the world. Caring for the whole person becomes a doorway to tell the story of Jesus and His Kingdom.

That Kingdom is what God is doing in the world through the Church, the Body of Christ. But it goes beyond the church,

---

[69] Geerhardus Vos, *The Kingdom of God and the Church* (Fontes Press 2017 reprinting of 1903 First Edition), 44.

[70] John Piper, *Providence* (Wheaton: Crossway Books 2020), 68.

focusing disciples outward to God's love for the world. Paul tells us in Colossians 1:20 that God's purpose in salvation was to reconcile all things to Himself through Jesus, "having made peace through the blood of His cross; through Him, I say, whether things on earth or things in heaven." Ultimately, God's work will bring heaven and earth together. Sickness and healing are rough sketches of this greater, final work.

Loving people by caring for the body is not just a sweetener for the gospel; it manifests the gospel. As theologian Geerhardus Vos put it, "The physical is not to be despised, but is to be appreciated…as the natural and necessary instrument of revelation for the spiritual."[71] The physical world reveals spiritual realities. We can make disciples who are learning how Jesus is Lord of these realities. This is why Jesus frames the Great Commission with the words, "All authority has been given to Me in heaven and on earth" (Matt 28:18) as well as "I am with you always, even to the end of the age." (Matt 28:20).

The Kingdom of God is "already" because it is happening in the present. But the Kingdom of God is also "not yet." Until Christ comes, a spiritual battle is taking place. This is not just invisible but manifests itself in physical ways–both in our bodies and in society. Therefore, disease and death won't be fully defeated until Christ returns to make everything new. And while the Lord often enables us to witness substantial healing, we will not have perfect healing or total success in healthcare ministry before He returns.

---

[71] Vos, *The Kingdom of God*, 33.

Questions for reflection:

I have argued that healing and salvation are neither separate nor identical. Do you agree? What was your understanding before reading this chapter? Can you live with healing and salvation in tension as I've described?

Have you seen sickness treated as sin? What were the consequences?

Have you seen bodily healing point to the bigger story of the Kingdom of God? Where and how?

CHAPTER 6

Saving Bodies and Saving Souls

Some years ago, as a mission, SIM refocused its purpose to "making disciples in communities where Christ is least known." Field leaders began to assess ministries–including health ministries–against this refocused purpose. One of them, a leader in an African country with established hospital and community ministries, struggled to understand how these ministries fit into this refocused purpose. It seemed to him that the doctors and nurses were caught up mostly in medical care, with little thought of the needs of these other communities. This led to conflict with the doctors and nurses, who felt unappreciated, and peripheral to mission decisions.

Mission leadership is often focused on church planting since the church is at the heart of God's program for blessing the nations of the world. It is not just mission leaders who wrestle with this question of how healthcare ministries fit with planting healthy churches. A survey of missionary healthcare workers in 2011 found that 38% believed their sending organization would prefer them to stop doing medicine and begin to focus entirely on other types of work![72]

Caring for the body has value. Matthew summarized his work in Galilee by saying, "Jesus was going through all the cities and villages, teaching in their synagogues and proclaiming the gospel of the Kingdom, and healing every kind of disease and every kind of sickness."[73] There is weight and significance to caring for the sick because Jesus did it.

On the other hand, ministry to the body must care for the whole person, like Jesus did. Complete healing moves the individual toward God's purpose in creating him or her. Whole persons are not independent of God, so whole-person healing must address meaning and hope. This means caring for the soul. How do we balance the physical and spiritual needs of the people we care for?

Health and salvation each carry weight and are integrally connected. Some say that physical and spiritual ministries are equal partners, similar in weight and importance. Others claim that ministry to the body is the means of getting to the *real* ministry (to the soul). They see medical ministry more like "bait" for evangelism. Is

---

[72] Webmaster. (2013, October 1). *Re-imaging medical missions: Results of the PRISM survey.* Missio Nexus. https://missionexus.org/re-imaging-medical-missions-results-of-the-prism-survey/
Also see Strand, M. A., Paulson, E., & Myrick, T. (2015). Characterizing the global context for cross-cultural healthcare work by regions of the world. Christian Journal for Global Health, 2(2), 23–38. https://doi.org/10.15566/cjgh.v2i2.78

[73] This same sentence is repeated by Matthew in 4:23 AND 9:35, indicating its importance. In between these bookends are the teaching (Sermon on the Mount, chapters 5-7), and healing (chapters 8-9) narratives.

this an either-or situation? No. But then how should we balance them? How should we set priorities?

I want to make the case that while bodily and spiritual ministries are both important and valuable, there is an ultimacy about spiritual priorities. The word *priority* conjures up all sorts of scary notions in our minds. *Priority* can imply urgency, significance, or precedence. It can also mean "right of way" or main concern. We may secretly fear that the ministry of healthcare (and our significance) doesn't matter much.

To illustrate how the salvation of body and soul work together, let's do something a little different. I invite you to join me in two thought experiments. Let's begin in the town and district around Capernaum, Jesus' headquarters in Galilee. Let's imagine two extremes.

Thought experiment #1: What if Jesus healed everyone?

What would Jesus' ministry have been like if He had responded to all—not just some—of the physical needs around him? What if He had healed everyone who came to Him around Capernaum? Imagine what that would've been like. Those who were sick would certainly have been rejoicing. There might have been dancing in the streets. Perhaps small dust clouds would have been kicked up amid the shouts of joy and worship. Jesus would have attracted quite a crowd of followers wanting to receive miraculous healing. Would they not have grown demanding, though? It's easy to imagine the scene taking a dark turn. The crowd might have grown so large and persistent that they would have restricted Jesus' movements from place to place.

Even if healed for a while, people would eventually have fallen sick again. Jesus did not give them resurrection bodies, even when He healed miraculously. They would still be susceptible to disease because death, like sin, is universal. Would they have turned on Jesus in their anger and despair? Eventually, they would face physical death and judgment. What of their rejoicing then?

The crowd's desire for bodily healing did become a problem for Jesus. In the early days of His ministry, He was faced with increasing demands for His healing from the residents of Capernaum and the surrounding localities:

> *When evening came, after the sun had set, they began bringing to Him all who were ill and those who were demon-possessed. And the whole city had gathered at the door. And He healed many who were ill with various diseases, cast out many demons; He was not permitting the demons to speak, because they knew who He was. In the early morning, while it was still dark, Jesus got up, left the house and went away to a secluded place, and was praying there. Simon and his companions searched for Him; they found Him, and said to Him, "Everyone is looking for you." He said to them, "Let us go somewhere else to the towns nearby, so I may preach there also; for that is what I came for." And he went into their synagogues throughout all Galilee, preaching and casting out demons.* (Mark 1:32-39).

Jesus focused on the root of the problem, without ignoring the symptoms. He chose not to set up a healing ministry in town (like Simon may have wanted Him to). He continued to move to other places, preaching as well as healing. He did something more sustainable in the long run. He did not bring in the Kingdom immediately but allowed His work of redemption to change the world gradually, like yeast working in bread.

Think of your community. What would happen if you could suddenly heal everyone around you? What if everyone was looking for *you*? How would you respond?

You may recall in Chapter One I described my own idealism that the church would be such salt and light that communities would change. Let's push this experiment to the extreme. What if we hoped (as an ongoing thought experiment) that Jesus would transform the culture of Capernaum, restoring *shalom*? To restore *shalom* Jesus would have had to end violence, adultery, lying, oppression, stealing, and covetousness. He would have had to bring in the Kingdom all at once. He didn't choose to do this.

The Kingdom of God does not rest primarily on the removal of suffering or brokenness but on the removal of sin. Redemption *first* transforms people from the inside, giving them a new heart, Kingdom, and citizenship. It prioritizes the inner, spiritual need to change the direction of our lives. As Jesus becomes King, He changes us and then changes the world through us. That which is heavenly gives direction to that which is earthly. The soul, not the body, must therefore take priority. The prophet Daniel describes it succinctly: "Heaven rules."[74]

Our experiment to prioritize healing is not working well. Focusing on complete physical healing doesn't bring in the Kingdom of God. Our Capernaum district is left with broken people, disappointed that Jesus did not do enough for them. The culture has yet

---

[74] Daniel 4:26

to be transformed, because, in our eagerness, our experiment left out the key ingredient: salvation from sin.

Jesus prioritized the root causes of brokenness: the sin that separates us from a holy God and thus also from each other. Bodily healing is only temporary until we receive new bodies. Even Lazarus, raised from the dead, lived to die another day. Since preaching God's Word is the key to this new life, Jesus prioritized the ministry of the Word over bodily healing. The gospel is the power of God for salvation to everyone who believes (Romans 1:16).

Jesus wept for Lazarus. Out of love, God truly cares about the suffering and death of men, women, and children, and demonstrated that love repeatedly. The miracles of healing show the character and intentions of the King. But the King brings in the Kingdom progressively, not all at once. Until He returns, we will still have some crying, mourning, pain, and death. Jesus cares about those things, and so should we. But we must make His priorities ours. We must love people by caring for their physical needs but also allow Him to use us to turn them to Himself and reorient their lives to God's purposes.

Detour: Healthcare ministry and the "Prosperity Gospel"

Let's continue to explore the implications of our first experiment. If we could somehow have made everyone physically well, what would this communicate to the world? We would become instantly popular, touted as highly "successful." We would be called miracle workers.

So many would demand our services that making time for listening and learning from patients would become challenging.

Building relationships would likely take a back seat to our success. Our behavior would tell others that our core mission is healing bodies, not making disciples.

Patients will only thank us and the system we represent if our health work does not point people to God. They may consider themselves fortunate, or just lucky. The spiritually inclined might bless the saints or angels; others might cling to superstitions. Some would honor the deities or idols they trust in. All these responses deny praise to God, the actual healer. Healthcare ministry without a God-ward orientation robs the Lord of the praise due Him. It can also become more about us as medical practitioners than Him.

Incorporating gospel words and conversations in healthcare allows us to challenge patients' false notions about illness. Human beings make meaning of disease and suffering, looking for ways to explain and relieve it. We continually seek to make things turn out well for ourselves and manipulate the unknown to our advantage. Anthropologists describe this as *animism*, a worldview that underlies all cultures and religious systems of the world (except vital Christianity). The thinking goes, "When I am ill, I won't get better unless I pray, chant, wear amulets, consult the shaman, or perform a certain religious ritual."

The "prosperity" or "health and wealth" gospel is a modern equivalent of animism but with a Christian veneer. This "gospel" says that if I do something for God (pray, have faith, be good, go to church, give money), God will reward me. It is a way of manipulating God rather than bowing to His sovereign purposes. It puts human beings and our selfish desires in the place of God. It is a false and deadly gospel.

The Lausanne Movement for Global Missions warns against Prosperity teaching this way: "We reject as unbiblical the notion that God's miraculous power can be treated as automatic, or at the disposal of human techniques, or manipulated by human words, actions or rituals."[75]

When we as Christian professionals expect dramatic results through medicine *itself*, we, too, are trusting something less than God. We violate our chief purpose: to glorify God and enjoy Him forever. We may find ourselves inadvertently teaching "Prosperity" by directing attention away from the glory of God and focusing only on bodily health.

SIM missionary doctor and Christian ethicist Tim Teusink tells of his surgical mentor, Dr. Al Snyder, at Kibogora Hospital in Rwanda. He claimed his life verse was Isaiah 42:8, where God says, "I will share my glory with no man." Tim explains, "If a patient said Al cured him, Al would quote this verse and attribute healing to God who had a purpose in healing the person. I've never forgotten that."[76]

The root problem of man's brokenness and sickness is sin, and without a radical solution to the problem of sin, we are powerless to bring wholeness. Only Christ can give that wholeness, and His way is radical: the way of the cross. Prosperity teaching has taken root in many places around the world, promising much but unable to deliver.

Disciples who know and obey Jesus, including the Christian doctors and nurses serving in the world's hardest places, should

---

[75] Jay Hartwell (2014, November 15). *A statement on the Prosperity Gospel.* Lausanne Movement. https://lausanne.org/content/a-statement-on-the-prosperity-gospel

[76] Dr. Tim Teusink, personal communication, used with permission

work to turn people and churches away from Prosperity teaching. This turning will help shape cultures for God's purposes. In this way, the "Prosperity Gospel," centered on mankind, will be replaced with one centered on God.

Thought experiment #2: What if Jesus chose not to heal physically?

Without being irreverent, let's consider the other extreme. What if none of our Capernaum residents experienced physical healing? Given His compassion, it's hard to imagine Jesus not healing people physically. But what might it have been like if Jesus concentrated solely on the preaching of the Word without the miracles of healing?

The words of Jesus are life-giving, so there would still have been rejoicing, but perhaps not the same intensity that the people experienced when receiving His word and His miracles *together*. At first, the little clouds of dust may not have risen as high. If Jesus chose not to do miracles, His words would still have been effective, because the gospel is the power of God for salvation (Romans 1:16). His words were sufficient to transform lives.

Jesus didn't "need" to show His authority by miraculous signs. He didn't use miraculous signs as bait for the "real" ministry of the Word. He was motivated to heal because of His character and the nature of the Kingdom of God. His love compelled him to heal. He demonstrates that "real" ministry *is* to the whole person, to restore human beings to the wholeness of God's image. In combining preaching and healing, Jesus modeled a ministry of words and deeds for us, married together, and expressed in love. And while

Jesus cared for the whole person, He always kept the right priorities: first our relationship to God and then to others.

The gospel does not change people without changing their lives. We don't "trust Jesus" in our hearts without a whole-of-life change. The power of the gospel expressed in love changes our outward lives, including our bodies and our relationships with others. Jesus transforms whole people and our response as His followers must be to give our whole life to Him. Faith without works is dead, being alone.[77]

In other words, Jesus makes disciples, not just converts. How do we recognize disciples? First, they yield to Jesus. Then they love others sacrificially. "For the whole law is fulfilled in one word, in the statement, 'You shall love your neighbor as yourself.'"[78] Ultimately this kind of love means obedience to *all* that Jesus commanded (see Matthew's Great Commission, especially Matthew 28:20).

So even if Jesus had not healed physically, He established a community of God's people who were transformed from the inside, freed from sin to serve God with full hearts. The lives of this community would have changed. These changed lives would begin to express the grace of God to others in the community, and by their good works demonstrate the goodness of God. The change would eventually be physical, not spiritual only.

Jesus makes us His disciples, with lives directed toward holiness and obedience. There should be no believer or church that does not impact the world in love. The church is called the Body of Christ precisely because it *is* His loving, physical presence in the world.

---

[77] James 2:17

[78] Galatians 5:14

The church, as the community of God's people, is to show forth the character of the King through gospel words and good deeds.

Even if no one is physically healed, the change Jesus brings in lives eventually results in various kinds of healing—from the soul to the body. Healing may result simply through disciples obeying the Word of God. While God in His sovereignty may choose not to heal a certain affliction, He frequently heals in response to answered prayer. Healing may follow from our wise choices, or through doctors and nurses who have studied hard and have the skills to care for those suffering.

One missionary tells us how his wife, a doctor, made disciples while visiting a neighboring country in Africa:

One of [her] highlights was to work with the young graduate doctors, saying "I consider it a privilege and honour to work alongside the expatriate missionary staff and the young doctors from Congo, Burundi, Chad, and Niger. Using Google translate from French to English, my broken Hausa, and a translator when available, I managed to do ward rounds with these bright young graduates who all speak French! We laughed, cried, prayed with patients when permission was granted, deliberated on the patients' management, and struggled with the suffering we saw as we attempted to treat our patients and counsel their families. Working from the stance that we treat but God heals in this low-resource facility, we saw many of our patients walking out of the hospital healed and well! Sadly, we also saw deaths, with

> *many coming too late. The mentoring was definitely a two-way process as I learned as much from them as they from me!"[79]*

God expects His Kingdom to permeate beyond individuals and churches. Vos explains that the Kingdom of God is "intended to pervade and control the whole of human life in all its forms of existence. This is what the parable of the leaven plainly teaches. These various forms of human life each have their own sphere ... There is a sphere of science, a sphere of art, a sphere of the family and of the state, a sphere of commerce and industry."[80] There is a sphere of healthcare as well.

Sadly, it seems too common to find churches that avoid the world and have little impact on the culture around them. Jesus says, "You are the salt of the earth; if the salt has become tasteless, how can it be made salty again? It is no longer good for anything, except to be thrown out and trampled underfoot by men."[81] Believers or churches that are insulated from the world are tasteless; they can't resist the corrosive forces of the world and don't contribute much to the transformation of the culture.

Vital ministries such as church planting or disciple-making should instill a love for the community in the church. Since we are whole persons, we can't expect a "soul" ministry without a physical expression. Jesus loves whole persons and whole communities; He sends His disciples to be the "light of the world." (Matt 5:14). Believers in church's love others by engaging with the culture, yet

---

[79] Prayer letter, May 2022, names withheld for confidentiality – used with permission.
[80] Vos, *The Kingdom of God and the Church*, 83.
[81] Matthew 5:13

they are different enough to make a difference, directed more by Scripture than by culture.

Jesus builds his church by making disciples who create communities (churches) that shape the communities around them. He gathers them together to build them up and then sends them out into the world to serve God and others.

We obey Jesus by making disciples and planting churches. We may not personally be church planters, but we can *plant a heart for the mission in its entirety*. Those with a heart for God's mission will love the church and also love organized mission efforts or institutions. Both church (gathered) and mission (sent) are vital to Jesus' work on earth. He uses us to change a few who begin to shape the world together with other believers. Our upward orientation towards God inspires our outward orientation to the suffering world.

Healthcare is an example of such service, and thus is a legitimate and often crucial part of the mission of the church, especially when the communities we are reaching are broken physically and are susceptible to diseases stemming from poverty, injustice, and abuse. A hospital can have this kind of mission if it has not lost this bigger vision. And healthcare mission should not be confined to institutions such as hospitals. Community disease prevention and health promotion efforts complement the care offered in hospitals. When we broaden our thinking about health, we will find that the church has much to contribute, especially by encouraging and participating in community-based efforts.

The beauty of a healthcare ministry is that God's love is demonstrated physically, in this world, not just in theory. Love is acted out, not idealized. The ministry to the body demonstrates the Kingdom of God's arrival. That Kingdom is not far away in heaven or set apart in churches, or only a future hope. It is not religious talk but actual, objective reality. It is the gospel lived out, with the power to change lives. That is what we are part of when we touch lives with healthcare!

Living out and proclaiming the gospel to the nations is our ultimate priority because it is Jesus' priority. Such ministry focuses us on God, who does not take us out of the world but rather sends us into the world with a new heart and orientation. As individual disciples and churches, we express that gospel heart by caring for individuals and communities with Jesus' compassion.

Getting our priorities straight

I've taken the liberty to paint two extreme, non-biblical pictures of salvation. The first experiment was all about physical healing and the second was an attempt to minimize it. Both are caricatures of the ministry of Jesus.

The first experiment reminds us that healing without salvation is temporary. It is right and good to relieve present suffering but not a long-term solution; it doesn't bring about all the changes God intends for human beings. It cannot change the heart. Christian healthcare is meant to be part of the broader mission of God to transform the world by changing hearts.

> **Healthcare ministry focuses us on God, who does not take us out of the world but rather sends us into the world with a new heart and orientation.**

The second experiment reminds us that salvation is still salvation even without physical healing. It will eventually lead to physical healing (either in this life or the next). God's words are "healing to your body and refreshment to your bones."[82] Healing of individuals, by God's grace, will eventually change communities, as we will see in Chapter Nine when we focus on the church. When Jesus inaugurates the Kingdom, He does so through whole-of-life transformation. He does not just make private converts or people who only come to church. He makes disciples.

So Christian healthcare ministry must marry together words and deeds, but always with an understanding of the ultimate priority of gospel words. Why? Because this is how Jesus makes disciples and changes the world.

This is why our understanding of the Kingdom of God—the gospel's big story--is essential. If the Kingdom is something immaterial, removed from the world at the end of the age, then it is hard to see how healthcare and church planting work together. But if the Kingdom has a material dimension (both now *and* in the future) then every ministry directed by Jesus has a role in bringing in the Kingdom. Can we reach a point where healthcare workers and church planters share a common vision to glorify God on the earth by enabling men and women to flourish and bless the world? God uses churches made up of Christ-centered disciples as his instruments to do this. Healthcare ministries are part of God's grand plan to build the Kingdom and shape the cultures of the world alongside healthy churches. Healthcare ministry does not stand alone but is one part of an integrated work of God to shape the world according to His purposes.

---

[82] Proverbs 3:8, Legacy Standard Bible

Our struggling African field director eventually left his position, in disappointment and brokenness that he was not able to bring healthcare ministry and mission onto the same page. God provided another director who was able to do so. He engaged the doctors and nurses, who took time away from their responsibilities to consider the integration of healthcare and mission. They recognized that they had been ministering out of their own narrow perspective, without much care about how they fit into the bigger picture of SIM's country vision. They found ways to help the church participate more intentionally in God's mission to bless underserved and unreached communities. This change enabled more synergy between efforts in healthcare and church planting.

So as healthcare workers, let's not work independently but rather join with Jesus in prioritizing discipleship, evangelism, and church planting. We'll consider in the next chapters how to do that.

Questions for reflection:

How do you set priorities for spiritual ministry when physical needs are so pressing?

Think of your community. What would happen if you could suddenly heal everyone around you? What if everyone was looking for *you*? How might you align your purpose with Jesus' purpose in and around Capernaum?

PART III

Aligning God's Purpose with Healthcare

CHAPTER 7

Healthcare Ministry and Making Disciples

Galmi Hospital is an SIM mission hospital in Niger on the edge of the Sahara Desert. Like many busy mission hospitals, it receives inquiries from physicians who want to serve but are concerned about the dangers of burnout. Some ask if they might be able to spend half-time in the hospital and half-time doing "ministry" outside the hospital in church or community. Others say that treating patients is a ministry in itself.

Missionary doctor Charles Fielding proposes a "Biblical Model for Missions" that brings healthcare and the gospel into homes. The author works in a context where public witness for Christ is restricted, so he emphasizes home-based outreach. He stresses the importance of discipleship but is skeptical about ministry in the hospital setting, with its multiple demands and time pressures.[83]

---

[83] Fielding, C., *Preach and Heal: A Biblical Model for Missions* (Richmond, VA: International Mission Board, 2008).

These examples raise the important question: what is a healthcare ministry? When does healthcare become *ministry*? You remember Yvonne (Chapter Two) also had a colleague who felt that the "real" ministry was bringing gifts and teaching the Bible to prisoners. We understand evangelism and Bible teaching as ministry, but is healthcare ministry "real" ministry?

The Apostle Paul tells us there are many kinds of ministry but the same Lord.[84] Ministry is not confined to those who serve the church by preaching and teaching. Jesus distributes various opportunities for service through the Holy Spirit. Some of us are called to ministry in healthcare. Healthcare ministry is compassionate care of the whole person. It focuses not only on alleviating suffering but also on helping provide meaning, seeking to share the good news of salvation from sin and restoration to wholeness in Christ. It means entering into the patient's world, listening, and loving in such a way that I can speak the truth to them—not just loving that I can diagnose Addison's disease or find an effective short-term TB regimen. It may even mean entering into their suffering in some way. Not every patient encounter will afford an opportunity to share the good news of the gospel. But every encounter must somehow connect their world with the love of Christ. And loving a person means I will have a passion that he or she becomes whole by knowing Christ, the source of all life and health.

Healthcare ministry doesn't isolate "spiritual" ministry from "physical" ministry, since we care for the whole person. Teaching the Bible to prisoners is ministry, but it does not become a healthcare ministry just because the minister is a doctor or nurse. Likewise, care for the body alone does not make it a healthcare *ministry*.

---

[84] See 1 Corinthians 12:5

Pastor and physician Dr. Martin Lloyd-Jones said, "Too many practitioners know more about some detail in the anatomy or pathology of a person than they do about the person himself. While we may talk more of, and pay lip service to, the concept of 'the whole man' and 'the complete patient,' we must be very careful that in fact and in practice we do not forget him."[85]

> **Healthcare ministry is compassionate care of the whole person. It not only alleviates suffering but helps provide meaning and shares the good news of salvation from sin and restoration to wholeness in Christ.**

We have seen that gospel ministry flows from the love of God for a broken and sin-soaked world. Serving Christ in healthcare is more than humanitarian service, which may be sacrificial but not directed to Christ. This love for our neighbors (patients, staff, and community) motivates us in Christian healthcare to see others flourish, especially by experiencing the fullness of life in Christ. Healthcare ministry has both individual patient care and community health in view since God's Kingdom transforms both.

My wife Clare and I served with our four children in Nepal in the 1990s under the International Nepal Fellowship (INF), which signed five-year agreements with the government of Nepal for healthcare and development. As a development agency, the INF greatly improved community health and livelihoods. However, the pressure to demonstrate development results to the government threatened to undercut our gospel efforts. We can sideline

---

[85] Lloyd-Jones, *Healing and the Scriptures*, 45.

the gospel in development or community health, just as we can in bedside care.

Does this more comprehensive scope of ministry mean more work? No. It helps us define the work and thus set boundaries, including Sabbath principles. Missionary doctor Jim Ritchie has written a helpful monograph on boundaries in healthcare. He points out that boundaries are God-given. "We human beings are not given that authority [over life and death], but we are given limited skills and abilities to heal."[86]

A clearer definition of healthcare ministry also makes the necessity for teamwork more obvious. After counseling, Cindy (Chapter Two) was much better prepared to work on teams, since she began attending to her relationships with colleagues and patients, rather than being driven by her inner needs. Clarity about her ministry made her boundaries more manageable. She was not "driven" to overrun her margins by unconscious motives. Healthcare ministry is about modeling the life of Christ for others, both patients and staff. Jesus starts by changing us. Cindy saw that attending to her inner self enabled her–and the team–to find more joy in the journey. This—and the establishment of her personal boundaries—began to change the team's culture, making the team itself healthier.

Missionary doctor W. Ted Kuhn shares his own experience of finding boundaries in the midst of overwhelming needs. He was in a remote village in Central America with a small medical team after a devastating hurricane. He describes countless needs, physical and emotional. A long line of patients was waiting for his small team

---

[86] J. Ritchie, *Boundaries for Healthcare Missionaries: God Honoring Structure for a Thriving Life of Service* (MedSend Publication, 2022), 4.

from the early morning. They pushed through to see 150 patients in a single day in the scorching heat. Kuhn writes:

> When the sun began to set, I noted that the line looked no shorter than it had in the morning. To our dismay, as we packed our supplies to leave, people cried and pleaded with us to stay a little longer, to see them, their child, their wife, or their mother. My heart broke. The pastor of the village leaned over to me and said, "Don't be distraught. The people who received care are satisfied. Those who did not receive care are not better, but they are no worse than before you came."
>
> It is good to remember that we are not responsible for their sickness. Life is a fatal illness! By God's grace, we assist some, but the needs will always be far too great. God never intended us to bear everyone's burdens. At the end of the day, we commit everyone—those who are seen and those who are not seen—into His care. That is where the burden belongs.
>
> In our early years in South Asia, we provided patients with self-retained medical records. This obviated the need for a complicated medical record system in a country where the most common male name is Mohammed, and most married women are called Begum. This worked well, and virtually no one lost their records. It took on average five days of standing in line to be seen as a new patient. However, once you have a chart and an initial exam, you could return any day for medicine refills or for a doctor's checkup with only a couple of hours' delay.
>
> One day, as I was triaging patients in line, a man stepped up to tell me that he was an "old" patient, but he did not have a medical record. This surprised me, as no one ever lost their record.

As the story unfolded, it became clear that we had never attended to this patient. He had waited with many other patients under the shade of the mahogany grove outside the clinic fence for several days without ever getting into the clinic. Unable to stay longer, and needing to attend to his rice crop, he returned home. His illness resolved along the way.

Now, he just wanted a recheck to make sure his illness was completely cured. He assured me this happened all the time. Many people would come to the clinic, but, unable to get in because of the line, they returned home to find their illness was either much better or completely resolved. Astonished, I turned to the crowd of more than five hundred waiting patients, and asked, "Is this true?" Many people verified that if you waited under the mahogany trees, your illness would resolve with or without seeing the doctor. That day, I understood I was not one of the only two doctors in the village. I was not even the senior physician. The Holy Spirit was at work, and it pleased Him to accomplish His will with or without my help.

In His pleasure, He sometimes allows us to participate in his plan of healing and redemption. He uses the prayers and intercessions of His saints (and sometimes missionary doctors) though we may be unaware what is occurring. But even if we cannot see all the patients in hurricane-ravaged Central America or the masses of South Asia, ultimately all patients are His. We need only to commit them to His hands and trust that He will do what is best for each and every one.

Now, decades after the incident under the mahogany trees as I arrive at a clinic site in the early morning and there are too many patients to care for that day, I walk slowly through the crowd. I touch or shake hands with as many as I can. I pray that each may have their spiritual eyes enlightened. I pray they may have an opportunity to see the gospel at work through the care given to others; through the prayer offered to all; through the unity and love of the team; and through the peace of resting in the sovereignty of God. I silently pray for each one, knowing that this day may be the closest they ever come to the Kingdom of God. I commit them into his capable hands, which is where they belong. I care for as many patients as I can, and at the end of the day, I pray that God has used me for His glory. The rest who did not get medical care are no better off. Yet, they are not worse off for my being there. I pray that the only One who can meet their needs will work in their lives, and that this day He will draw near, touch them, and hear their cries.[87]

Why disciple-making at the core?

Healthcare ministry involves both compassionate medical care and evangelism. Making disciples not only adds these together but multiplies them. Disciple-making is the heart of healthcare, not something separate. It includes evangelism, for sure. But the core verb in Jesus' Great Commission is to make disciples. This means inviting others to know Jesus Christ and building others up to grow in Him. Disciples love God and their neighbors well. Making disciples in healthcare ministry aligns us with the mission of God for the world.

The New Testament word for disciple (*mathetes*) refers to a person who follows and seeks to learn from another. Luke 6:40

---

[87] Excerpted with permission from Kuhn, W.T., *Heal in Imitation of Christ: Conversations on Medical Missions* (Trusted Books, 2014), 121-124.

reminds us that a disciple seeks to become like his teacher. "In this way, discipleship is about modifying one's entire lifestyle."[88]

Disciples are those who follow Jesus and obey Him, not a special class of believers. Disciples in healthcare ministry will take every opportunity to share the good news of the gospel of Jesus with all who do not know him. But, in addition to the words of the gospel, disciples will know the heart of the gospel. Disciples will connect with staff and patients such that the fragrance of Christ will be evident. Disciples become salt and light in the culture–preserving, changing, and shaping it.

Working closely with the healthcare team is a precious opportunity to shape the lives of those we work with. Rather than a separate spiritual program divorced from work, making disciples this way enables each person on the team to develop Christ-like character and use his or her gifts to minister to others.

The Saline Process[89] teaches healthcare workers to be witnesses of Jesus Christ at bedsides and clinics around the world. One mission hospital decided to train the entire staff, not just doctors and nurses at the bedside. A guard, who previously had seen his job as gatekeeper and "tough guy," was transformed. He was excited to see how he fit into the hospital's mission to make Christ known. He began to see his role as not keeping people out but inviting them in. As he received patients at the front gate, he welcomed them to a community showing Christ's love! Even guards can be disciples and make disciples.

---

[88] Byrley, C., "Discipleship" in D. Mangum, D.R. Brown, R. Klippenstein, & R. Hurst (Eds.), *Lexham Theological Wordbook* (Bellingham: Lexham Presss, 2014).

[89] *Saline — IHS Global.* IHS Global. https://ihsglobal.org/salineprocess

Not all our patients or staff will be Christian; not all will be disciples. But in healthcare ministry, we work in teams with apprenticeship models. Teams are ideal for sharing not only the techniques of medicine but also the soul of medicine—changing hearts through healthcare. Our aim is more than good patient care or the transfer of information. We share Christ through what we say and how we connect with others.

Disciples become salt and light in their own spheres of influence, beyond the clinical setting to home, family, community, and nation. Their influence will extend to their own churches and communities. And even if God calls them to a different team or location, they will have the opportunity to continue to shape the world, because their hearts have been changed.

The bottom line of ministry: disciples whom Jesus so transforms can't help but glorify Him by what they do and say. Whatever their current "job" is, their lives can be examples of sacrificial service to others. Can you begin to get excited to see even one person's life transformed, fully engaged with God as a disciple of Jesus, and using his or her knowledge of healthcare to address some of the deepest challenges of the culture?

This is the way that Jesus' Great Commission to make disciples connects to the cultural mandate. Making disciples is His appointed means to bring the blessings of the Kingdom of God to the world. Disciples do not extract themselves from the world but go *into the world* for Christ. This means making a difference in the culture for Christ, not conforming to culture or being against it.

Jesus confronts the brokenness and sin of this world with His own righteous Kingdom. He is ushering in a Kingdom whose citizens, as described in His Sermon on the Mount, recognize their spiritual need, mourn over the world, and are gentle, hungering and thirsting for righteousness.[90] He commands us to "seek first His Kingdom and his righteousness."[91] His people shine the light of Christ on the injustice, violence, and greed of this world; Jesus works through them to make changes. Healthcare ministry is a strategic way to follow God's plan. The key is making disciples.

What does making disciples mean for us?

Since God has called us to make disciples as we care for the sick, our character and culture matter a lot. Jesus said, "A disciple is not above his teacher, but everyone when he is fully trained will be like his teacher."[92] It is not enough that we as teachers do the right things; we must have Jesus shining through us. God calls us not just to our work, but to our relationship with Jesus.

Dr. Martyn Lloyd-Jones tells us, "So the great call to us is that we should become whole men *ourselves* and thereby be in a position to deal with 'the whole man' when patients come to us. Let us really understand what is basically wrong. Let us go beyond what technical medicine and the most modern therapy can offer and point men to the Way, the only way in which they can become *whole* men."[93]

This is easy to say, but what does it mean in practice? Let's explore what it means for us—professional teachers and mentors—to be disciples ourselves.

The son of one of our physicians serving in Africa was waiting for his dad to play a game of UNO with him during his lunch break

---

[90] See Matthew chapters 5-7
[91] Matthew 6:33
[92] Luke 6:40
[93] Lloyd-Jones, *Healing and the Scriptures*, 51.

from the hospital. The family had recently arrived at the mission hospital from a medical practice in the West, where he had practiced happily for years. But the doctor had no appetite for a game or conversation; he went to his own bedroom. There would be no UNO today.

Later, his wife asked sensitively, "What is going on? Why so despondent?"

Her husband explained, "This morning I've had more children die than I've seen in all my medical practice back home. What am I doing here if I can only help so few? Am I enough for this ministry?"

Serving cross-culturally as a missionary can upset our deepest assumptions about who we are and our place in the world. Like this doctor, we may ask ourselves: "Am I not called to heal people? How can I function with such limited resources? How do I meet the overwhelming need? How can I cope with the fragility of life? What do I do with all my sorrow?"

Why does healthcare care sometimes not *feel* like a ministry? Why is it so common to feel overwhelmed, undervalued, afraid, and often frustrated? The vicarious trauma we experience as healthcare providers can affect us profoundly, especially the ethical dilemmas that experts call moral injury. Hope may be found not simply by changing the circumstances of our ministry but by examining the margins and boundaries we set for ourselves.

"I have to decide between burnout and moral injury," complained a missionary surgeon. "If I do everything that is asked of me, I will burn out. It's inevitable. No one can continue to work like this. But if I don't do everything that is asked of me, I will feel morally injured. I will be guilty of having failed someone at a time of great need. And if I have to decide between burnout and moral injury, I'll pick burnout every time. For me, being a medical missionary is a direct path to burnout."[94] Ritchie explains, "Overwork and burnout may be the most common preventable reason healthcare missionaries leave the field and do not return."[95]

I began to lose a heart of joy during my first years in Ethiopia when so much seemed ambiguous and things didn't go according to my plans. My identity as a missionary and physician was tied up with trying to accomplish my own plans rather than trusting the Lord to work out His. I had placed human "*doing*" ahead of human "*being*." I was becoming what Christian writer Gordon MacDonald describes as a driven person, not a called person.[96]

In my case, I knew my position in Christ in my head, but I was driven by wanting to perform, to be seen as the best. My vocational call was somehow not integrated deeply enough with my identity in Christ. The Lord used the anxiety and frustration of missionary healthcare to soften my heart. Strangely enough, I was more open to sharing my vulnerability and admitting my brokenness when I was hurting. You too may find yourself in a similar situation, overwhelmed. Take heart! It is a process! And an opportunity!

MacDonald writes, "Driven people often project a bravado of confidence as they forge ahead with their achievement-oriented life plan. But often, when it is least expected, adversities and obstructions conspire, and there can be personal collapse. Called people, on the other hand, possess strength from within, a quality of perseverance and power that are impervious to the blows from without."[97]

---

[94] Ritchie, *Boundaries for Healthcare Missionaries*, 3.
[95] Ibid., 53.
[96] Gordon MacDonald, *Ordering Your Private World* (Nashville: Thomas Nelson, 2003), 53.
[97] Ibid., 58.

For me, learning to be a disciple of Jesus meant learning to rest in Him when my work seemed insignificant. It meant not neglecting my most important relationships in a vain attempt to make my work count. Ultimately, it meant less about me and more about Him.

Theologian Dr. Richard Lints warns us that our culture has taken a subjective turn.

> *The testimony of evangelicals centers too frequently on what Jesus means to them and what the Holy Spirit is doing in our lives. We speak too little about what Jesus has accomplished in His own life and death, too little about the ways in which the Holy Spirit is connected to Jesus and to the furthering of His Kingdom. We emphasize the one who has the faith rather than the one who is the object of faith.*[98]

To put making disciples at the core of healthcare ministry means that *I* must be growing as a disciple. *My* unconscious assumptions, mental map, or worldview, need to be challenged. Christian anthropologist Paul Hiebert explains, "In mission settings, we should examine not only the worldviews of the new converts but also of *ourselves* as missionaries, for in the past we have often been shaped more by modernity than by the gospel."[99] [italics mine]

Jesus uses mistakes, disappointments, and conflicts in healthcare ministry to call us back to Himself. William Perkins, a beloved Puritan writer, distinguishes our "general calling" to Christ from

---

[98] Lints, R., *The Fabric of Theology* (Grand Rapids: Eerdmans, 1993), 335.

[99] Hiebert, P.G., *Transforming Worldviews: An Anthropological Understanding of How People Change* (Grand Rapids: Baker Academic, 2008), 231.

our "particular calling" to our vocation. Our calling to Christ always takes the lead and shapes our particular calling in healthcare.[100]

Like Cindy, you may discover blind spots where you need help. You want to find your way back to a heart of joy. She found healing through relationships that helped her recover her identity in Christ. Relationships are key. Family, friends, professional counselors, and mentors all enabled her to begin to thrive, not just survive.

"Born a man, died a doctor?"

Writing to physicians in the 1980s, Dr. Martyn Lloyd-Jones portrays the doctor himself:

If I were asked to mention the most serious of these [temptations] I would say that it is a proneness to objectify everything, or in other words, to take a 'detached view.' I suppose this is to some extent inevitable. If a medical man were continually to allow himself to be affected emotionally by every case he meets, it is fairly clear that he could not continue long in practice... While that is all perfectly understandable, it does, however, lead to a particular danger. It becomes a fixed habit of mind. The doctor has so objectified himself that he never faces up to himself and to his own life at all.

Somewhere in Pembrokeshire a tombstone is said to bear the inscription, "John Jones, born a man, died a grocer." There are many whom I have had the privilege of meeting whose tombstone might well bear the grim epitaph: "... born a man, died a

---

[100] William Perkins and C. Matthew McMahon, *Glorifying God in Our Jobs* (Crossville: Puritan Publications, 2015).

doctor"! *The greatest danger which confronts the medical man is that he may become lost in his profession.*[101]

How does our identity in Christ shape our calling to healthcare? For starters, we can see that while Christ cared for the physical and spiritual needs of many, He established limits. As we found in Mark 1:32-39, He did not try to heal everyone looking for healing in the district of Capernaum. As much as He had compassion on (and healed) those with physical needs, His driving purpose was to preach to a wider audience.

After a grueling term overseas, one of our doctors asked for help with burnout. A colleague in the home office asked him, "What really motivates you? *Why* do you do what you do?"

> **"The greatest danger which confronts the medical man is that he may become lost in his profession." – Dr. Martyn Lloyd-Jones**

"Because of the need!" he explained quickly.

The colleague replied, "That's the wrong answer."

The doctor didn't respond for a long time.

Continuing, the colleague declared, "Need motivates you to many good things, but if it all depends on you, then, of course, you will burn out. The real answer is the glory of God."

"I'm going to have to think about it," the doctor whispered.

Like this doctor, how do we keep from becoming lost in our profession? How do we keep from dying as doctors (and healthcare

---

[101] Lloyd-Jones, *Healing and the Scriptures*, 14.

professionals) instead of living on a mission to reveal the glory of God?

As medical professionals, we are shaped in our training and experience by a secular perspective that minimizes or even excludes God and His goal for humanity. The profession itself can become our identity, so we narrow our focus to the body only, the here and now, and avoid conversations about meaning and purpose. Our profession can shape our lives more than we like to admit.

Tournier wrote, "If the mind of the doctor is filled exclusively with scientific preoccupations, if he thinks of nothing but microbes, chemical doses, or psychic complexes, the patient will never speak to him of the questions which torment him and which concern the meaning of his illness, rather than its mechanism."[102]

Am I a doctor, surgeon, or nurse who happens to be Christian, or am I a Christian who happens to be a doctor, surgeon, or nurse?

William Perkins says, "The true end of our lives is to serve God in serving man."[103] Healthcare ministry is more than a professional calling; it is a sacred calling. The sacredness does not stop with evangelism but continues with discipleship. Making disciples is the Lord's powerful means of transforming the world and healing the nations.

Creating margins and avoiding burnout are not scheduling issues but heart issues. Making disciples while caring for patients guards us against two errors. The first is the fatalistic lie that because the needs are so great, we cannot make much

> **Healthcare ministry is a sacred calling.**

---

[102] Tournier, *A Doctor's Casebook in Light of the Bible*, 15.
[103] Perkins and McMahon, *Glorifying God in Our Jobs*.

difference. Making disciples multiplies our efforts. It builds the capacity for God to move through others.

The second error is the optimistic lie that we can do everything by ourselves. This certainly has been a temptation for me, with my perfectionistic, workaholic tendencies. I have had to learn that I am not called to *all* the good things that may need to be done. Jesus sets before us just enough for one day at a time. I rely on my wife and others to help me from going beyond healthy margins. Making disciples builds their capacity and also helps me from taking on things that others could or should be doing. It's a potent safeguard against burnout.

Making disciples helps align healthcare ministry and the larger purposes of God, so I hope we can avoid these two extremes. To repeat them, the one says, "I'm not a part of what God is doing here, so I have no value." The other extreme says, "I'm responsible for everything (evangelism, church planting, medicine, community, etc.)." If the first extreme places too little worth on me, the second one places too much.

Cindy found that a new perspective changed the quality of her work as a healthcare provider. She came to see that healthcare ministry is not about the amount of pathology we treat but about how we treat the people with the pathology. Showing God's love (the quality of our work) takes precedence over the quantity of our work.

Achieving quality and compassionate care requires teamwork. And teams are made of people, some of whom are not yet disciples and others who are. Healthcare ministry is about making disciples, both of patients and staff. At the core, it is about the birth and growth of these disciples. The way we act creates a team culture, and that culture demonstrates Christ in word and deed.

In the long run, a Christ-centered health team culture can impact the church and community. We have seen that the church, the Body of Christ, is God's instrument to bring salvation and healing to communities where unrighteousness and human brokenness prevail. In the next chapter, we'll look back at how God has used his church to do that from the beginning.

Questions for reflection:

How would you define healthcare ministry? What has been your own understanding of disciple-making? What is your own role in making disciples?

Do you struggle with work-life balance? Who might help you establish wise boundaries?

CHAPTER 8

Church, Compassionate Care, and Culture

I was once meeting with a group of older pastors in Mozambique. They had been young when the gospel first entered their village. I asked them, "What sort of difference did the gospel make to your people? Did you see changes?"

Their response was firm and enthusiastic. "Yes! Before the gospel came to us, our families lived in fear. Hatred abounded. Even though we were all the same clan, no one could be sure he would not get a spear in the back when venturing outside the house!"

"How did the gospel change things?" I asked. I won't forget their answer since it sums up the gospel so well.

"The forgiveness we received from Jesus changed our whole culture!"

This chapter is about how the church began to shape the culture, and especially the culture of healthcare. We want to examine the extent of this impact and the reason for it. How did God use the church to care for the sick? What was the church's understanding of ministry to the sick? What can we learn from the past to help us build a healthcare ministry shaped more by the gospel than by modern assumptions?

Believers laid a foundation of care for the sick which developed during the Roman Empire (until the fifth century). Despite being small and persecuted, the impact of the church was profound and continued to mature until the dawn of modern scientific medicine (nineteenth century) and beyond. The gospel not only transformed healthcare but also helped form our modern views about sickness.

First and second centuries: Compassionate care is born

The Roman view of persons was utilitarian; if someone was not useful to society, he was not considered valuable. This perspective created scenarios of suffering that we might find unfathomable today. Christian medical historian Gary Ferngren writes, "Compassion was not a well-developed virtue among the pagan Romans; mercy was discouraged, as it only helped those too weak to contribute to society. In the cramped, unsanitary warrens of the typical Roman city, under the miserable cycle of plagues and famines, the sick found no public institutions dedicated to their care and little in the way of sympathy or help. Perhaps a family member would come to their aid, but sometimes even close relatives would leave their own to die."[104]

---

[104] Ferngren, G.B., "A new era in Roman healthcare," *Issue 101 | Christian History Magazine* Christian History Institute, 2011, 6. https://christianhistoryinstitute.org/magazine/issue/healthcare-and-hospitals-in-the-mission-of-the-church

Roman Christians, however, were encouraged to visit the sick and help the poor, and each congregation organized ministries of mercy. Mercy is something they had experienced and thus wanted others to experience. Believers served others because Christ had done so. Christ came to serve, not to be served like the gods of the Romans.

Christian ministry to the sick was a ministry of caring more than curing. It was based on love for the whole person. Christians developed relationships with people in need, not merely souls that inhabited bodies. Church Father Tertullian described how central our bodies are to salvation; he wrote of the flesh as the "pivot [hinge, fulcrum]" of salvation.[105] "The ministry of medical care in early Christianity began as a church-based diaconal, not professional, ministry. Unskilled, ordinary people provided it with no medical training. Yet, the church created in the first two centuries of its existence the only organization in the Roman world that systematically cared for its destitute sick."[106]

The early ministries of believers to the sick harmonize with the definition of healthcare ministry we reached in the last chapter: healthcare ministry is compassionate care of the whole person. It focuses not only on suffering but also on its meaning, and it seeks to share the good news of salvation from sin and restoration to wholeness. These believers shared the gospel in both word and deed. Tertullian claimed, "It is our care of the helpless, our practice of loving kindness that brands us in the eyes of many of our opponents. 'Only look,' they say, 'look how they love one another.'"[107]

---

[105] *Tertullian, de resurrectione Carnis, 8 – 9.* https://www.vatican.va/spirit/documents/spirit_20000908_tertulliano_en.html

[106] Ferngren, "A new era in Roman healthcare," 12.

[107] Stark, R., *The Rise of Christianity* (San Francisco: Harper One, 1996), 87.

At the same time, Ferngren emphasizes that the care for the sick was not considered a special healing ministry. Christians did *not* promise physical healing or miracles. There was no separate ministry to the body. Caring for the sick was "an important part, but only a part, of the general philanthropic outreach of the church, which included widows and orphans, aiding the poor, visiting those in prison, and extending hospitality to travelers."[108]

Medical professionals in the Roman Empire were schooled in rational, Greek medicine. The medicine of that day, based on the humoral theories of Galen, was not particularly effective.[109] Physicians served those with money and status. While believers at that time were not against professional care,[110] the church's ministry to the sick was not grounded in the medical profession. Their care was born out of compassion for human beings made in the image of God, not the medical theories of the day.

What lessons can we learn from the ministry of these early believers to the sick? Their ministry developed out of their understanding of the gospel and the imitation of Christ.[111] Certainly, as His followers, we want our ministry to do the same. And while we

---

[108] Ferngren, G.B., *Medicine and Healthcare in Early Christianity* (Baltimore: Johns Hopkins University Press, 2009), 46.

[109] Wooten, D., *Bad Medicine: Doctors Doing Harm Since Hippocrates* (Oxford University Press, 2006), 8-13.

[110] Ferngren, *Medicine and Healthcare in Early Christianity*, 13.

[111] Christoffer Grundmann explains that Church Father Gregory of Nyssa taught that the imitation of Christ (see 1 Cor 11:1 for example) was more than attempting to copy Jesus' example, but living a life translucent for Christ as the Lord. It is Jesus' life through believers that touches people today. Salvation is corporeal (bodily) not just soulish.
See Grundmann, C.H. (2018) Christ as Physician: The ancient Christus medicus trope and Christian medical missions as imitation of Christ. *Christian Journal for Global Health*, 5(3), 3–11. https://doi.org/10.15566/cjgh.v5i3.236

minister with much more technical expertise today, we mustn't forget that *charitable ministry to the sick grew out of the life of the church.* This is important for us, since we may not think of the church when we consider health care. Yet today's culture of care for the sick has been shaped by the gospel more than by Galen.

Third century: Care moves beyond the churches

God led the churches in the third century to minister to others outside the church, regardless of faith. As individual Christians began to minister to the sick and poor, churches began to organize this assistance. Ferngren wrote of this model:

> *The administrative structure of the local church (ecclesia) was simple but well suited to the supervision of charitable activities that relied largely on voluntary activity. Each church had a two-tiered ministry composed of presbyters [elders] and deacons (see Acts 6:1-6), who directed the corporate ministry of the congregation. Deacons, whose main concern was the relief of physical want and suffering, had a special duty to visit the ill and report them to the presbyters: "They are to be doers of good works, exercising a general supervision day and night, neither scorning the poor nor respecting the person of the rich; they must ascertain who are in distress and not exclude them from a share in church funds, compelling also the well-to-do to put money aside for good works."*[112]

---

[112] Gary Ferngren, *Medicine and Health Care in Early Christianity*, 114.

A devastating epidemic spread in the Western Roman Empire in 250 AD and lasted 20 years. The cause may have been plague or smallpox. At its height, 5,000 people a day were dying in the city of Rome itself, apart from the devastation of rural areas.[113] Supplication was made to the Roman gods to learn what might stop the plague, but public officials otherwise did nothing to prevent the spread of the disease, treat the sick, or even bury the dead.[114]

Sociologist Rodney Stark wrote in *The Rise of Christianity*, "At a time when all other faiths were called to question, Christianity offered explanation and comfort. Even more important, Christian doctrine provided a prescription for action."[115]

Pagan Romans pushed sufferers away, throwing them onto the roads even before they were dead, hoping to escape the fatal disease. Bishop Dionysius tells us there was not a house in which at least one person hadn't died. But heedless of danger, the believers attended to their needs and ministered to them with the love of Christ.[116] Despite the absence of effective medical treatment, caring Christians treated the sick by drawing near them, offering a cup of cold water, attending to their physical needs, and sharing the comfort of the gospel.

Some sick were healed, and others died but departed this world trusting Christ for their bodily resurrection. Many of these caring believers also became infected, essentially offering their lives for others.

---

[113] Stark, *The Rise of Christianity*, 77.

[114] Ferngren, "A new era in Roman healthcare," 11.

[115] Stark, *The Rise of Christianity*, 82.

[116] Ibid., 82

The love of Christ motivated early Christians to minister beyond their own family, tribe, or church. Charity was extended to the community as a whole, especially to those who could not help themselves. This kind of sacrificial love cannot be bought. Healthcare ministry was not motivated just by the needs of the sick but by the love of God.

During the first three centuries, it was not possible for Christians who were undergoing persecution to establish permanent institutions for the care of the sick. Yet, churches became hubs for the care of the sick in hundreds of cities throughout the Roman Empire.[117]

A century later, the Roman Emperor Julian complained that the moral character of Christians and their love for strangers was causing the growth of the church. He wrote, "The impious Galileans support not only their poor, but ours as well; everyone can see that our people lack aid from us."[118]

Ministry to the sick was a powerful witness for Christ and gradually began to transform the Roman empire. Stark asserts that the magnitude of the movement to Christ during the epidemics contributed to the fall of Roman paganism, which could not confront the crises socially or spiritually.[119]

What can we learn? This ministry to the sick, shaped and nurtured by the gospel of Christ, saved many from death, both physically and spiritually. *The gospel did not just change individuals but also churches, creating a new outward orientation towards the poor and sick.* It set the stage for the fourth-century, where ministry to the sick became even more organized and outward-focused.

---

[117] Ferngren, *Medicine and Health Care in Early Christianity*, 145.

[118] Ibid., 84.

[119] Ibid., 94.

In caring for the sick, the churches aligned with God's purpose of bringing the good news of Jesus to the poor and healing the brokenhearted.[120] Let us learn how to work with churches to orient care outwards towards the poor and sick.

Fourth-century: Birth of hospitals

While many in our modern world may point to Christianity as an enemy and destroyer of culture, the historical evidence is exactly the opposite. Historically, Christian ministry to the sick has done much to transform the world and even change the culture of medicine. Bishop Basil of Caesarea ("the Great"), honored for his work in solidifying the doctrine of the Trinity, is widely credited with founding a new Christian institution, the very first hospital, in AD 369.[121] Some monastics led lifestyles of self-denial, which seemed to reinforce Plato's teaching that the body is evil. Bishop Basil, by contrast, created a new type of Christian monastery that focused not just on the salvation of its community of monks but on the physical care of the sick and poor.[122]

While Christians made early efforts to reach out to the sick, some were concerned that the medical profession opposed God's will. Greek physicians had developed a rational approach to health, based on observation, anatomic studies, and drug experiments.

---

[120] Isaiah 61:1-3

[121] Miller, T.S., "Basil's House of Healing," *Issue 101 | Christian History Magazine* Christian History Institute, 2011, 13. https://christianhistoryinstitute.org/magazine/issue/healthcare-and-hospitals-in-the-mission-of-the-church

[122] The Buddhist Indian King Ashok the Great (3rd century before Christ) made an edict ("Rock Edict II") to build institutions for medical care for needy humans and animals, but his reign lasted only 50 years. See Mark, J. J. (2023). The Edicts of Ashoka The Great. *World History Encyclopedia.* https://www.worldhistory.org/Edicts_of_Ashoka/

"But Christians were suspicious of medicine because it put its faith in human *logos* rather than in the Divine *Logos*, Christ."[123] Basil countered this thinking, "arguing that God gave Adam and Eve agriculture to feed their families, weaving to clothe their nakedness, and the *logos* of medicine to heal their diseases."[124] Basil played a significant role in convincing Christians that medical science was a gift from God, not a pagan deception. This helped remove doubts about working with physicians.

> **The gospel did not just change individuals but also churches, creating a new outward orientation towards the poor and sick.**

The word hospital is rooted in the Latin word *hospes*, meaning guest. Basil's unique institution had "guest houses" for pilgrim travelers, places for the aged and sick, and refuge for those suffering from leprosy. Basil felt that those with leprosy deserved care, despite the fact that physicians had no idea how to treat it. There were also houses for physicians and nurses. "The community of men and women at the Basileias (House of Basil) dedicated themselves both to worshiping God and to assisting the sick (whom Basil's physicians attempted to heal) and travelers needing a clean, safe place to stay."[125]

Ferngren informs us, "The hospital was, in origin and conception, a distinctively Christian institution, rooted in Christian concepts of charity and philanthropy. There were no pre-Christian

---

[123] Miller, "Basil's House of Healing," 15.

[124] Ibid., 15.

[125] Ibid., 14.

institutions in the ancient world that served the purpose that Christian hospitals were created to serve, that is, offering charitable aid, particularly health care, to those in need."[126]

What can we learn and apply from fourth-century Christians? Chiefly, *Christian healthcare has a particular orientation to those who are the least in society's eyes.* As a distinctively Christian expression of the gospel, the hospital had a particular concern for the poor and marginalized. It began to formalize ministry beyond what individual churches could do alone. Healthcare professionals in cross-cultural service follow an ancient Christian expression when we organize ministries for the poor and brokenhearted.

Fifth century and beyond: Hospitals as a signature Christian ministry

Over the centuries, Christian hospitals evolved from charity houses for the poor to more modern institutions. Historian Sharon James notes, "By the fourteenth century, England alone, with fewer than four million people, had six hundred hospitals; France, Germany, and Italy had even more. The Benedictines alone were responsible for more than two thousand hospitals."[127]

> **Christian healthcare has a particular orientation to those who are the least in society's eyes.**

In *The Influence of Christians in Medicine*, J.T. Aiken writes that "Western Medicine, from the fourth-century AD to this present day, has owed a great debt

---

[126] Ferngren, *Medicine and Health Care in Early Christianity*, 124.

[127] James, S., *How Christianity Transformed the World* (Glasgow: Christian Focus, 2021), 132.

to Christianity and to individual Christians for the maintenance of its tradition and practice."[128] The building of Christian hospitals emerged in the Middle Ages in the 12th century. Secular authorities were challenged and stimulated by the church's example in the countries served by these hospitals. By the 18th century in Europe, "so greatly did the number of hospitals increase that it has been called the 'age of hospitals.'"[129] Christian hospitals introduced "a new attitude toward the sick, an attitude of pity and a desire to help, [which] was quite new in that it extended to strangers and, still more remarkable, to the poor."[130]

As Christian ministries, these institutions became a signature of the integration of body and soul. Christians did not merely explain the Bible to their cultures, they demonstrated it, thus shaping and changing culture. Hospitals were unique Christian institutions in serving those who could not pay back.

Christian ministry was not confined to hospitals. In the early church, deacons and deaconesses cared for the sick. The profession of modern nursing, for example, grew up out of the vision of a German pastor Theodor Fleidner, who established a hospital to train deaconesses to provide nursing care as a Christian ministry. Florence Nightingale became one of his more famous graduates.[131] Individual Christian physicians and nurses have shaped healthcare up to and through the period of scientific medicine (which began about 1850). (We will learn more about the modern period in Chapter 10).

---

[128] Aitken, J.T., Fuller, W.C., Johnson, D., *The Influence of Christians in Medicine* (London: Christian Medical Fellowship, 1984), vii.

[129] Ibid., 17.

[130] Ibid., 17.

[131] James, *How Christianity Changed the World*, 137.

A prominent historian of medicine, Henry Sigerist, wrote that "Christianity introduced the 'most revolutionary and decisive change in the attitude of society toward the sick,' giving sick people 'a preferential position' in society that they retain to this day."[132] Christian author Vishal Mangalwadi reminds us that while Greek, Roman, and Islamic civilizations produced professional doctors and surgeons, these cultures could not create a culture of care.[133] Are you energized to be part of a tradition that has made this sort of positive impact on the nations of the world? I am!

Questions for reflection:

If you had a minute in an elevator to explain to someone how Christians over the centuries have shaped healthcare, what would you say?

Has Christian healthcare shaped the churches in your community? How?

How might an understanding of the history of the church's care for the sick help your local churches engage more fully in ministry to the whole person?

---

[132] Ferngren, "A new era in Roman healthcare," 12.
[133] James, *How Christianity Changed the World*, 128.

CHAPTER 9

Health, the Church, and the Mission of God

I agreed to mentor the lead physician in one of our African mission hospitals. The hospital seemed to be thriving, busily serving a large rural community. But Tom (not his real name) said, "Our doctors are discouraged."

"Why? What are the reasons behind it?" I replied.

"They feel that headquarters doesn't really appreciate them anymore," Tom said.

Knowing SIM's strong commitment to medical ministry, I was surprised. Continuing to dig, I said, "Tell me about that."

Tom answered, "Last year our country director came and basically told us that the hospital no longer fits in the mission's vision for the country. He's a church planter. Since most of the local population has now become Christians, it is hard for him to see how the hospital does much more than care for their physical needs. Now that the church is more established, should our focus be elsewhere?"

Tom knew that some mission boards had backed away from hospital care in favor of church planting.

It was discouraging for Dr. Tom and his colleagues to think their own mission no longer believed in their work. In Chapter Seven, we said that healthcare ministry means making disciples. Tom's director was looking at another picture: planting healthy churches. When the church is more established in a certain area, is the healthcare ministry's or hospital's purpose completed? Is it time to move on?

The answer to this question depends a lot on how we connect healthcare ministry and God's mission. If we exclude the church, assuming that healthcare ministry *alone* will accomplish the mission, we are in danger of bypassing God's instrument for shaping the world: the church. But what kind of church are we talking about? Will that church care about its mission to the poor?

The word "mission" can be defined as the sending into the world of the Son or the Spirit by the Father for the purpose of salvation, or the work of churches or mission agencies to preach the gospel and establish a gospel presence (the church) among the nations. But while God accomplishes His work through the church, the purpose of His work is not confined to the church. The mission of God has the whole creation in view, not just the church.

The mission of God is ultimately about the revelation of God's glory to all creation. Jesus is restoring humankind to His purpose, to bless the nations and the world. That Kingdom transformation is present "now" and "not yet." God reveals Himself through the church to the world, transforming individuals and changing communities. Mission, then, is not just about our activities or church, but about transforming the world according to God's good purposes. It is present now and will be fulfilled completely in the future.

I am using the word "ministry" more modestly, as a service to accomplish the broader goal of God's mission. Bible teaching is ministry, just like healthcare or sports can be ministries. All these ministries are, in a sense, strategies that contribute to the wider goal of the mission of God. Aligning ministries with the church's work creates synergy for accomplishing the purposes of God.

Healthcare ministries that focus primarily on evangelism may find their value questioned once people have come to Christ and churches are established. This seems to be the case with Dr. Tom's mission director. But healthcare ministries that define their mission more as discipleship can contribute to both the initial stages of church planting (evangelism) as well as the later stages of church growth and outreach (disciple-making). Christian healthcare ministry is a gift to the church to help shape the world for Christ, and the church is essential to the fruitfulness of healthcare ministry.

Jesus' Great Commission in Matthew 28:18-20 aligns *ministry* (evangelism and discipleship) together with the *church* (baptizing and teaching them) to carry out the *mission* (Jesus with us to accomplish what He has commanded):

> *All authority has been given to Me in heaven and on earth. Go therefore and make disciples of all the nations, baptizing them in the name of the Father and the Son and the Holy Spirit, teaching them to observe all that I have commanded you; and lo, I am with you always, even to the end of the age.* (Matthew 28:18-20).

The Great Commission is the means God uses to accomplish the larger mission of the Kingdom of God. That's why discipleship is critically important; it is the key command in the Great Commission. Discipleship is not a stand-alone ministry; disciples become part of churches to participate in the mission of God in the world.

The prophet Habakkuk says, "For the earth will be filled with the glory of the LORD, as the waters cover the sea."[134] God is on a mission to glorify His Son among the nations. This grander, more global view helps integrate our church-planting ministries with our healthcare ministries. It also points back to a much earlier expression of the good news, God's promise to Abraham to bless the ethnic groups of the world (Genesis 12:1-3).

Missiologist Andrew Walls emphasizes this bigger, more corporate view of mission. Walls points out that the mission is not just about discipling *individuals* but about discipling *nations*.[135] "The Great Commission is not just a broadcast of the Word of God through these communities, but penetration into the distinctive ways of thought, kinship, and shared mental and moral processes of the community."[136] Through disciples, the Word of God becomes flesh in the community and in all the ethnolinguistic peoples of the world. As long as there are communities and nations where Christ is not known, there are opportunities to make disciples who will reach out to them, sharing the gospel and planting groups of disciples (churches). The gospel is God's means of transforming culture.

---

[134] Habakkuk 2:14

[135] Walls, A.F., *The Missionary Movement in Christian History* (Maryknoll, New York: Orbis Books, 2005), 48.

[136] Ibid., 51.

Aligning ministry and mission

The newly formed board of directors of one of our mission hospitals in West Africa was given the essential task of defining the mission and vision of the hospital. The question came up as to who the beneficiaries were. Was our target community simply the patients who showed up for care? Or should we be thinking more broadly about a particular impact the hospital wanted to have? To what community or constituency were we, as a board, fundamentally making promises?

> **The mission is not just about discipling individuals but about discipling nations.**

I asked my fellow board member, "If God gives time and energy, do we want to have a particular emphasis on serving poor communities?"

This godly brother, eager to see a strong emphasis on evangelism at the hospital, said, "I don't see that we have time or resources to reach communities."

I replied, "True enough for now; we are not ready yet. But could our hospital eventually be a resource for those communities, teaching or training believers in churches that want to reach them?"

"I'm not convinced that is the hospital's mission," he said.

I respect my brother on the board greatly. He sees the "mission" as primarily evangelism. Evangelism has motivated many mission hospitals over the last century and a half. In West Africa, for example, an SIM surgeon founded another hospital decades ago which has maintained a twin emphasis on surgery and evangelism. The Jesus video is being used extensively; people are finding Christ. But new believers are getting lost when they return to their village because of hostility to the gospel and lack of Christian fellowship. The answer to this dilemma is to work with churches to find a more comprehensive view of the "mission" that enables church and healthcare ministries to work together. Evangelism is essential but is part of a larger effort that extends to communities.

Healthcare and evangelism are each only a *part* of this broader mission of God. *Making disciples* is the key command in the Great Commission, but the disciples we make don't thrive without churches. Ultimately, the church—a community of disciples—is God's means of transforming communities and nations. The "mission" of healthcare is the same as the "mission" of the church: to make Christ known to the nations by making disciples. In that way, we participate in His Kingdom and transform culture. Making disciples is God's means of transforming the world.

This wider mission vision connects what we do in healthcare to churches and to the community. Without an appreciation for the bigger mission of God, we might begin to define our goal as meeting the needs of those who come to us, either physical or spiritual needs. But since these needs are endless, how do we set limits? The mission of God allows us to find our true north. Rather than just reacting to needs, we can begin to set a more meaningful course by linking up with churches to make disciples with a heart for the mission of God.

A healthcare ministry without this larger sense of mission is prone to only solve today's problems as patients come to us (or as we meet people in community health ministry). Meeting needs can trap us in a cycle of demand and activity. Alternatively, we can look at the bigger picture and proactively shape healthcare ministry with churches and local believers. This will help us better use limited resources to contribute wisely to the church's overall mission, participating with them in the Great Commission. God uses ministries of deeds and words together to accomplish His will.

How might healthcare ministries collaborate with churches to fulfill Christ's commission? We'll start first by looking at what each brings to the table. *Notice how each collaboration highlights the importance of making disciples.*

1. Healthcare ministries break down barriers.

In Southern Ethiopia the remote Bunna tribe did not easily extend trust to outsiders. However, the nurses who were able to deliver babies were welcomed into homes. We often find ourselves in low-trust cultures. Everything we do in healthcare can build (or destroy) trust. Genuine relationships break down barriers to the Word of God. Healthcare gives access to people's lives in an intimate way that other ministries sometimes cannot.

2. Healthcare helps focus attention on those who are lost and suffering.

Churches exist for worship and for building up believers to do the work of ministry. To do this, they must have something of an inward orientation. Mission efforts like healthcare are oriented outward towards the world and unbelievers. Both orientations are essential to the work of Christ's commission. Both are important in God's plan to transform the world. A ministry like healthcare can sustain a focus on the lost and suffering over an extended period of time. That focus can be strengthened when the healthcare ministry combines with other ministries to reach the world for Christ. The recent COVID-19 pandemic threatened to overwhelm healthcare systems during its first wave. Rather than turning inward, some churches in Africa and Asia began to ask themselves how to prepare for overwhelming numbers of dying people. Several of us in SIM developed a training module and videos in response to a request from churches in Zimbabwe, Kenya, and Bangladesh. The church leaders wanted to train those who would minister to the dying and also protect them from COVID. They developed church-based ministries that combined good science with good theology.

3. Disciples in healthcare ministry can catch a vision for the mission.

Not all disciples will become missionaries, of course. Yet all disciples are directed by Jesus to the mission of making Christ known and obeying Him in everything. In the 1980s, SIM Evangel Hospital in Nigeria developed a new family medicine residency training program. Australian missionary doctor Phil Andrew described the program in 1993, saying, "[SIM's] task now is training, and not just in the technical area. These committed Christian doctors live with us on the compound and we are involved with them as colleagues' day in and day out. We are now in a mentoring or disciple-making role, and this is a major switch. The type of people we now need [to recruit] in our hospitals are doctors with firstly a solid academic and professional background to enable them to teach effectively, and secondly a commitment to making disciples. People with these interests, combined of course with the usual requirements among SIM missionaries to Nigeria, namely flexibility, patience, sense of humour, willingness to work under the church, etc., are finding great fulfillment in their ministries in the medical department of ECWA [church]… We neglect the training of national health workers to the peril of the emerging church."[137]

4. Churches build up disciples over the long term.

There is a communal nature to discipleship; disciples are not formed in isolation from others. Health ministry teams make disciples, but the growth of disciples must not stop there. Healthy Christian communities build men and women through fellowship, preaching, and teaching of the Word of God. Churches are an essential part of the life and growth of disciples.

5. Churches are the key to long-term sustainability and change.

Hospitals and ministries that reach the poor have always needed some outside support to thrive. Remember that the church's early hospitals were built on a Christian culture of compassion. Compassion led to charity and generosity (the root of modern philanthropy). Ministries that care for those who cannot pay back will always need generous donors who value the work. The gospel is the root source of that generosity and sustainability, whether the resources are from outside the country or inside.[138] Local believers can also contribute to long-term leadership and governance of Christian healthcare ministries, which is even more important than financial sustainability. Churches and local believers can also play

---

[137] Phil Andrew, "Training Health Workers in SIM: The Quiet Revolution in Medical Mission Strategy" (Sydney), 1993

[138] Colossians 1:6 says, "This same Good News that came to you is going out all over the world. It is bearing fruit everywhere by changing lives, just as it changed your lives from the day you first heard and understood the truth about God's wonderful grace." (Col 1:6, NLT)

a vital role in closing or changing healthcare or hospital ministries that have fulfilled their God-given purpose.

> 6. *The church can also get a vision to love and support its healthcare workers.*

As emissaries of Christ in the marketplace and community, these workers can receive support and guidance from the wisdom of believers. What an encouragement to a young nursing student, for example, when she learns in church how crucial her ministry is to God.

What are the implications for healthcare ministry?

How do we make disciples with a view toward this broader impact of mission? Here are four suggestions. Let's take them one at a time.

> 1. *Intentionally instill a love for God's mission in the hearts of your fellow healthcare workers.*

Many young Nigerian medical professionals are beginning to go cross-culturally to unreached and underdeveloped communities in West Africa to make disciples. But in discussing the definition of *missionary* with some of them, I discovered they believed the term could not apply to themselves. In their view, *missionary* was a term applied to someone from the West who had traveled far and was supported by others back home. But truly, missionary is not defined by the source of income or distance from home but by a passion for making Christ known among the world's least-reached peoples, especially those who are marginalized and poor.

God has called us to serve in cross-cultural situations that are culturally distant to us, including those in foreign countries. Missionaries experience the costs of goodbyes, transition, fund-raising, and learning a new language. They serve at salaries often much lower than salaries back home. Local disciples who catch a vision of the mission of God may experience similar issues. They will make some of these same sacrifices (and sometimes bigger ones), whether serving in their own country or a remote one. It is these kinds of disciples whom the Lord will use to continue the work of mission both in healthcare facilities and beyond to communities that are physically and spiritually underserved.

2. *Address issues rooted in the culture and community with your colleagues.*

God calls some healthcare workers to focus their efforts on prevention and community health, while others are called to bedside care (which is a good thing) while *also* providing key support to community health efforts. Our role may not take us regularly outside the hospital or clinic but as we learn from patients about their lives, we will begin to identify some of the root causes of disease. We will learn how they think about illness and healing as well as their dreams for the future. These dreams and challenges will point back to the communities in which they live.

For those healthcare workers who are focused on community health, visiting individuals in the community and learning about challenges can help bring perspective to the diseases we see every day. We may find abuse, violence, lack of education, lack of basic hygiene, and many such trials present when God's *shalom* is absent. Our purpose is not to "solve" these problems but rather to begin to understand and pray about issues that are beyond us. God may give our local colleagues a vision of how to tackle them by partnering with local believers.

In his book *Let's Build Our Lives*, medical missionary statesman and teacher Dr. Dan Fountain describes twelve village men and women sitting under a tree with Pastor Simon.[139] The pastor tells them a story and asks God to help them in a discussion. Together, they identify things that were keeping them from experiencing the fullness of life Jesus came to give (John 10:10). This led to a conversation about sick children, lack of job opportunities, and HIV and AIDS. He encourages them to work together to tackle root causes rather than symptoms only. The discussion that follows begins to connect community problems with the meaning of illness, the place of spells or curses, and God's place in sickness. We need these sorts of discussions in our communities.

Disease care and community care are complementary. Stan Rowland, a missionary entrepreneur, has developed a constructive approach to community health called "CHE," or Community Health Evangelism.[140] In 1982 I worked with Stan for a short time in Uganda in a community health program. Physicians are often not prepared for community health, and the CHE model offers tools for this kind of work.

Our local healthcare colleagues may not have our technical training, but they can be more effective in connecting with those suffering in the community. As medical professionals, we can speak with a certain amount of authority and help our colleagues

---

[139] Fountain, D.E., *Let's Build Our Lives* (Brunswick, Georgia: MAP International, 1990), 7.

[140] Mahon, J. (2023, May 6). *What is CHE – Global CHE Network*. Global CHE Network. https://chenetwork.org/learn-the-strategy/what-is-che/

multiply their impact as disciples of Christ. Could you see yourself spending even one-half day monthly in the community with these colleagues? And if you are already working in the community, how might you partner with your local churches and other Christian healthcare ministries?

3. *Support churches in addressing illness and suffering in communities that need Christ.*

The Evangelical Church of Liberia (ECOL), a SIM-related church, has had the vision to reach out to remote and needy Muslim communities in Liberia for some years. Their leaders began praying and planning even when the church budget had no money for these activities. Nurses and healthcare workers who are part of ECOL have joined with non-medical believers in multiple, fruitful outreaches. They are building bridges with these communities by loving people through medical outreach and the gospel. Small groups of new believers have begun to form as a result. The mission hospital where these medical professionals work has an opportunity to partner with ECOL as a resource to help these churches address community needs.

Hospital budgets tend to be tight, but modest investments can make a big difference to community health efforts. Training can be one such modest investment. During the COVID-19 and HIV and AIDS pandemics, an SIM team trained churches that found their own financial resources, taking ownership of the ministry. Over the long term, it is not just money that sustains programs but vision and spiritual leadership. We saw churches take leadership during these health crises.

A Kenyan mission hospital has sent Kenyan resident physicians short-term to remote communities to give them a taste of healthcare missions. Some are beginning to return to those communities for the long-term. The Indonesian Christian Medical and Dental Association has had the vision to train Indonesian Christians to return to serve in former "mission hospitals" among poor communities. The Nigerian fellowship has developed a similar initiative. Churches are a vital part of such outreaches.

4. Partner with churches in mission outreach.

Paul Tournier argues that we must not say that medical professionals treat the body and that the church treats the soul. Both of them are part of a single reality! Both must work together. "From science, then, the doctor learns the mechanism of things, and from the Bible their meaning."[141] Let's be sure mechanism and meaning work together.

Increasingly, medical professionals from the West have been staying in service for shorter periods of time, even those committed to "long-term" missions. Issues of medical licenses, malpractice, and loss of professional continuity seem to make lifetime commitments more complex and costly. Our Western family systems are sometimes more fragile, so it takes longer to work through our dysfunctions to have healthy relationships. Lack of boundaries and burnout are important issues. Yet, unreached and underserved communities still abound. What is the future of healthcare missions?

While Westerners will continue to have an important role, partnering with churches will mean teaching and learning from

---

[141] Tournier, *A Doctor's Casebook in the Light of the Bible*, 35.

non-Western medical professionals. Modern medical training is available in some form in most nations of the world, and most nations have established churches and denominations that are beginning to send medical professionals into missions. Christian physicians and other healthcare professionals from these nations see the potential of serving the Lord through healthcare. Some have become effective cross-cultural missionaries. Doing healthcare ministry together gives the opportunity to disciple them and to be discipled by them.

Healthy churches will seek to reach groups of people who don't know Christ, and, often, we as healthcare workers can provide some medical care or teaching to assist them. Christian nurses and health workers are also members of local churches and often hold leadership roles. These local believers can help bridge the gap that is sometimes seen between the Bible and health.

Partnering with churches does not only mean working with nurses and doctors. At the bedside, chaplains can be a very important part of a team, listening and speaking to, praying for, and sharing with patients. Non-medical staff can also make a tremendous difference. In one hospital in Zimbabwe, discharged patients living far away are referred to pastors near their homes by text messages. These approaches integrate the gospel, church, and healthcare.

As healthcare workers serving Christ, our concern for the whole person will lead us to have God's heart for the whole community and the nation. Only the gospel will make a difference in the community and shape the culture in a God-glorifying, Satan-defeating direction. Churches are Christ's means of bringing the Kingdom of God on earth. Healthcare ministries must strive to collaborate with churches to make disciples who will obey Him in all that He commands.

Next, let's take a look at the broader mission of God through the lens of modern medical missions over the last two centuries.

Questions for reflection:

What is your vision of the mission of healthcare, and how does this connect with the mission of the church? Does anything make you doubt you can collaborate with churches?

How might you partner with churches and others to impart a heart for mission in those whom you work most closely with?

CHAPTER 10

Medical Missions and Healthcare Missions

During one of my visits to Malawi, I heard of a poor community living near Lake Malawi. They had a significant burden of ill health and yet no health facility. Several of their leaders met with our SIM Director to ask the mission to build a clinic. They knew the mission had provided clinics and medical care in other parts of the country.

The director asked, "Since you are Muslim, could you not appeal to friends in the Middle East to help you build a clinic?"

They responded, "Yes, we could get money from Saudi Arabia to build ourselves a clinic, *but we can't buy compassion!*"

The Malawi village leaders recognized the uniqueness of Christian medical missions. Over the last two centuries, medical and healthcare mission efforts have blessed the world with spiritual and physical healing. Many have found Christ through the loving care of nurses and doctors; suffering has been alleviated, and Christian medical and nursing schools have been founded. Entire communities have been impacted for good. But there is room for improvement. Non-biblical assumptions have challenged our best efforts.

In this chapter, we will consider how cultural assumptions have shaped these two centuries of medical missions, threatening to knock these efforts out of alignment with the mission of God. I will divide this time into two periods and suggest that each period has faced somewhat different challenges. The first period, or "medical missions," extended from the early 1800s to 1970. The second period, or "healthcare missions," continued from 1970 to the present. Each of these periods is shaped by its own distinctive cultural perspective.

The period of medical missions: the nineteenth to mid-twentieth century

The first period of medical missions began after William Carey, considered the father of modern missions, was sent from England to Calcutta in 1793. Medical mission historian Christoffer Grundmann tells us that the first medical missionary was Dr. Peter Parker, who arrived in Canton, China, in 1834. Dr. Parker studied both medicine and theology at Yale. His aim was to love the Chinese through medical care, preaching the gospel, and distributing tracts. His work in China began this entire period of medical missions, which lasted about 150 years. By the 1970s there was a shift in missions towards primary healthcare, which we will consider later as a second period.

Peter Parker inspired the formation of the Edinburgh Medical Missionary Society in 1841. It was created to identify and send medical doctors from Scotland to serve Christ around the world. The church's passion for world evangelization was evident at the founding of the Edinburgh Medical Missionary Society. During inaugural lectures, Rev. Jonathan Watson said, "The Medical Missionary ought to be deeply impressed, in every situation, and in all circumstances, with the fact that he is himself a Missionary of Jesus to the heathen."[142] Dr. George Wilson, in a lecture on the "Sacredness of Medicine as a Profession," said, "The patient's soul, as well as his body, is entrusted to his [the doctor's] charge; and he must aim directly at the former, as well as seek to reach it through the latter before he can attempt a cure."[143]

Historically, medical missions and modern medicine grew together. Enthusiasm for world evangelism developed in the nineteenth century, just as epoch-making discoveries in medicine were ushering in the age of scientific medicine. "It was this series of discoveries that aided the rapid development of medical missions."[144] Grundmann reminds us of anesthesia (1846), asepsis (the prevention of childbirth fever by Semmelweiss, 1847), and their application to surgery by Lister (1867). Names like Virchow (cell pathology, 1850s), Pasteur (1863), and Koch (bacteriology) are well-known to medical students. Later in the 19th century, these were followed by the discovery of the leprosy bacillus, the malaria parasite, and the bacteria that causes typhoid. X-rays were also discovered before the

---

[142] Watson, J., "The Duties of a Medical Missionary." *Lectures on Medical Missions: Delivered at the Instance of the Edinburgh Medical Missionary* Society (Edinburgh: Sutherland and Knox, 1849), 209.

[143] Ibid., 225.

[144] Grundmann, C.H., *Sent to Heal! Emergence and Development of Medical Missions* (Lanham: University Press of America, 2005), 45.

end of the century. Christian physicians and nurses were eager to share these advances in the global cause of the gospel.

Grundmann tells us that six physicians were sent to China in 1863. By 1925, there were over one thousand physicians, a similar number of nurses and midwives, and over five thousand local co-workers."[145] This represented about 10.5% of the total missionary personnel serving abroad.[146] "In January 1900, using imagery based on the then-common and cherished parallel between military imperialism and missionary activity, H. Lankester described medical missions as 'the heavy artillery of the missionary army.'"[147]

In the 19th century and for much of the 20th, medical missionary work was concentrated in hospitals, often started by a single physician, although clinics, dispensaries, and public health work were important, too. Western doctors and nurses, under colonial flags, went to serve remote and forgotten communities. Their passion was fueled by the *twin* desire to make Christ known among the nations and to offer modern healthcare to suffering populations.

Nigerian historian Yusufu Turaki shares an example of the power of medical missions, writing, "The contribution of the SIM medical work in Northern Nigeria was quite substantial and was the largest of all Christian missions. SIM was also the largest contributor in Northern Nigeria towards leprosy work and fighting eye diseases and blindness." He continued, "This ministry of mercy and caring was also a ministry of soul-winning and evangelism. It would be difficult to quantify the impact of medical work and services

---

[145] Grundmann, *Sent to Heal*, 150.
[146] Ibid., 150.
[147] Ibid., 150.

in establishing Christianity in the Sudan [Sub-Saharan Africa]. However, its influence and impact are observable facts...."[148]

The long-term influence of medical missions is suggested by a recent study that documents a "robust, positive association between proximity to a Protestant medical mission and current individuals' health outcomes" in India.[149] The authors connected contemporary health data with historical information on the location of mission hospitals. They attribute positive health outcomes to changes in hygiene and health habits.

Ferngren tells us, "At first, Protestants thought of it [medical missions] as mainly strategic, a means of gaining a hearing for Christianity in areas where mission work did not find ready acceptance... *Over time, medical missions tended to abandon efforts to use medicine in the service of evangelism and were content to make medical service an end in itself.*"[150] Certainly, this was not universally true, but how was this possible? How could evangelism begin to take a second seat? To understand, it will help to examine some of the assumptions underlying medical missions during this period.

Assumptions during this period of medical mission

The Christian Medical Dental Association holds an annual continuing education conference for healthcare missionaries serving abroad. Those who participate come from many nations. Several years ago, at one such conference, African surgical residents being

---

[148] Hudson, "Ministries of Compassion," 277.

[149] Calvi, R. and Mantovanelli, F.G., "Long-term effects of access to health care: Medical missions in colonial India," *Journal of Development Economics* 135 (November 2018): 285-303.

[150] Ferngren, G.B., Medicine and Religion (Baltimore: Johns Hopkins Press, 2014), 170 [italics mine].

trained and discipled through Christian residency programs across Africa were in attendance. They were asked during a presentation, "What is the ONE main lesson you have been learning in your residency programs?" The room was quiet as everyone waited for the response. Those present were eager to learn how these men and women would begin to set the pace as rising Christian leaders to meet Africa's vast unmet surgical needs.

The answer was shocking! A young resident spoke up for the group and replied, "The one thing we have learned is that the MOST important thing about surgery is that *work* is the most important thing."

They had learned well the silent message about the priority of work. They had "caught" an unspoken worldview assumption from their Western mentors. As a result, they were becoming as tired and burned out as other doctors. This is even more disturbing when we consider that these mentors were usually medical missionaries dedicated to serving the Lord. How could they have communicated that work is more important than our relationship with God? Like them, we can be very sincere yet blind to our own suppositions.

Christian anthropologist Paul Hiebert argued that cultural transformation takes place at three levels, from surface to deep.[151] On the surface are behavior and ritual (attend church, avoid tobacco, read the Bible). Beneath are beliefs (knowing Scripture, understanding how the world works). At the deepest level is the worldview (our basic understanding of reality, often unconscious or assumed). As we disciple others, we are shaping behavior, beliefs, *and* worldview.

---

[151] Hiebert, *Transforming Worldviews*, 316.

We, in turn, have been shaped, often unconsciously, by our own cultures. To help our disciples learn to integrate faith and medical practice, we must become students (and critics) of our *own* worldview as medical professionals. We communicate not just with the words of our teaching but also with our lives. The apprenticeship model of medical care is a powerful way of shaping behavior, beliefs, and worldviews. We unconsciously pass on the cultural assumptions—good and bad—that mold our understanding of our work.

What assumptions about work and ministry were active in this early period of medical missions? Doctors and nurses were strongly motivated by both evangelism *and* the newfound capacity of scientific medicine. These two powerful purposes could work together but in reality often produced discord. Such discord was evident when mission leaders saw medical missions only as a means of evangelism. Dr. Parker's experience in China is a case in point.

Because of Dr. Parker's success in practicing ophthalmology and the fame that ensued, he "could hardly find the time needed for proper and serious language studies."[152] Patient care demanded much of his time, despite his enthusiasm for evangelism. The leader of his American mission board, Dr. Rufus Anderson, was adamant that "We should give the people the Scripture, and organize our converts into churches–native throughout, self-governed, self-supported, self-propagating." Anderson believed a missionary should promptly leave when the church was fully organized.[153] He eventually dismissed Dr. Parker from the mission!

---

[152] Grundmann, *Sent to Heal!*, 64.

[153] Gulick, E.V., *Peter Parker and the Opening of China* (Cambridge: Harvard Press, 1973), 132-143.

Grundmann tells us that medical missionaries "constantly had to defend the validity of their medical practice as missionary work."[154] The lack of a coherent purpose for medical missions often led to conflict with mission leaders. Medical missionaries "tended to defend their work somewhat apologetically." He explains that they "hardly–if ever–succeeded in formulating and communicating the rationale for their own work in such a way that others could fully understand them."[155]

In formulating a defense for medical missions, these medical mission pioneers drew their understanding of reality from a world shaped by the Enlightenment. From about 1750 onward, people began to see the world as material and the body as a machine. The world of our senses became the "real" one, and heaven, revelation, and God became distanced (or not considered real). It's not difficult to see how medical professionals would come to see the world divided between body and soul—or medical care and evangelism.

The Enlightenment view of reality excludes meaning and purpose from physical care. This perspective dehumanizes people. When we no longer see human beings as whole persons created for a purpose, we undermine our own task as Christian healthcare workers.

Historian James Hannam contrasts this modern mind-body dualism with the unity of the medieval period. He wrote, "The central idea of the medieval worldview was that everything and everybody had a purpose. Nothing just happened. Nothing existed purely for its own sake. The ultimate governor of the universe was God, and He had endowed everything with a reason for its

---

[154] Grundmann, *Sent to Heal!*, 202.
[155] Ibid., 202.

existence."[156] This assumption helped launch the scientific revolution. "[Medieval Christians'] central belief [was] that nature was created by God and so worthy of their attention."[157] But *our* modern, naturalistic worldview puts the world in the center and removes God as the sovereign and good governor of all. In this worldview, there can be no larger purpose for human beings or their suffering.

Grundmann describes the dilemma of medical mission pioneers this way:

> *The structure and delivery systems of medical missionary work can best be described in terms of medical missionaries' efforts to replicate in an overseas setting the very medical practice and system [modern scientific medicine] they themselves were trained in. Their strong advocacy of scientific medicine, which in their own lifetime they had witnessed as able to do so much good, prevented their letting their own assumptions be challenged in the encounter with other cultures.... The rapid and effective advances in Western scientific medicine, which they greeted with obvious enthusiasm, gave them a false sense that their own work could only be increasingly successful and a pure blessing to everyone. They could not do otherwise, because they lacked the historical distance necessary for profound criticism. To take on that task is the privilege—and duty—of those who come after them.[158]*

---

[156] James Hannam, *The Genesis of Science* (Washington, DC: Regnery Publishing, Inc., 2011), 27.

[157] Ibid., 343.

[158] Grundmann, *Sent to Heal!*, 219-20.

During this first period of medical missions, the temptation was to be increasingly involved with the overwhelming physical need. It was not always clear how the medical work connected with the bigger story of the mission of God. The outcome was that, at times, the mission drifted from its calling.

I found my naturalistic assumptions challenged on the Tibetan plateau in 2001. I was part of a small group of Western Christian doctors and nurses invited to a remote village on the dry plateau. We took a bus until the road ran out and then carried our bedding, water, and gear up the steep inclines. A village monk welcomed us to treat villagers, suffering without access to modern medicine. Rain is very infrequent on the plateau, but the monk told us that it had often rained during previous medical visits by missionaries. The Buddhist villagers interpreted this as a sign from heaven. We arrived under sunny, blue skies. It seemed obvious there would be no rain during this particular stay.

We spent the next three or four days on the mountain consulting with the village people about common things (abdominal pain, joint pain) and uncommon (severe rheumatoid arthritis, tuberculosis, fatigue of unclear origin, etc.). Our limited formulary did not allow us to treat every condition, but, with permission, we prayed for each person in Jesus' name.

The night before we left the mountain, the heavens burst open! It rained so hard that we barely made it down the slick descent. Arriving home hours later, we were covered in mud. The monk told us afterward that it had not rained that hard in *seventy years*!

I had to force myself to ask, "Where does the rain actually come from? Did God send that rain or was it due to chance meteorological conditions? Did God work sovereignly through natural causes?"

It was painfully obvious that God loved these people so much, that He wanted them to know Him. He was pleased to show His power over creation by sending the rain. We learned later that several folks had been completely healed of serious illnesses! God had also shown them His power through healing.

We learned that these villagers were surprised that we listened to their responses when we asked questions! Without thinking, we had communicated their value as human beings made in the image of God, a God who heals. And while we were unable to share the gospel in words during our visit, others who followed afterward could do so. Many later came to faith in Christ. God communicated His gospel to them through gospel words and deeds. God was healing whole persons.

What story did this first period of medical missions communicate?

This first period of medical missions reflects the cultural reality of the nineteenth and early twentieth centuries. Modern people see reality as divided between the natural (secular) and the supernatural (sacred). This division can lead to a split understanding of mission: medical care is for the body and spiritual care is for the soul. This modern worldview encouraged them to fragment medical missions into the competing priorities of evangelism and healthcare.

Despite its limitations, this dualistic approach to medical missions has born fruit, both physically and spiritually. Individual healthcare workers have been incredible examples of sacrificial service and cultural influence. Tremendous institutions have grown up to help the poor and marginalized. My concern is that fragmenting the mission of God into two reduces the impact of the whole. A fragmented story loses its punch; it distorts the message.

Evangelism and healthcare are each part of a larger story; they are not meant to be separate or in competition.

Jesus' ministry communicated a whole story. The Apostle Mark tells us that the people listening to Jesus teach had not eaten for three days. Surely the spiritual ministry was uppermost on Jesus' mind, yet he told his disciples, "I feel compassion for the people.... If I send them away hungry to their homes, they will faint on the way." (Mark 8:2-3). His feeding of the four thousand this way demonstrated His seamless integration of the spiritual and physical aspects of life.

Here's how we distort the story. Our medical care for others shows that we value the body here and now, but our words seem to direct them to a different, future world. If we cannot make the connection between these two worlds, our hearers may be puzzled, asking, "Should I trust God now for my needs when He seems to be most concerned about another world? Why not rely on medicine and science?" Or, "Can I trust God for the future when He is not meeting my present needs?" Only the gospel story provides the link between present realities and future promises. The biblical story weaves the thread between the "now" and the "not yet."

We must communicate a coherent picture of humanity's place in God's plan to restore our broken world. Theologians Michael Goheen and Craig Bartholomew tell us that "in order to make sense of our lives, we depend on a story to provide the broader framework of meaning...Every part of our lives will always take its meaning from some larger story."[159] The grand story of the Bible enables us to find the meaning God intended for suffering and illness.

---

[159] Goheen, *The True Story of the Whole World – Finding Your Place in the Biblical Drama*, 2.

Without this grand story, we may inadvertently communicate that healing is *in the medical care itself* and that sickness and health are not God's concern or in His control. This reinforces the notion that healing is private, something I can buy or own. Without the grand story of the Bible, how will our patients connect their suffering with God's purposes for themselves and others? Health easily becomes divorced from His mission to restore the world.

Remember Yvonne in Chapter Two? Some of her co-workers saw ministry as spiritual work, and others as primarily medical. There was no shared story, and thus no clear vision or ministry purpose. The ministry of the hospital would have been stronger if the physical and spiritual work had been integrated with God's wider purpose in the church and the community. This would have allowed the community to grasp the story of how Jesus is working to bring about a Kingdom to change their world!

Medical mission work must start with recognizing the false assumptions that can undermine the work. The gospel story gives us a coherent, consistent message, from creation and the Fall to the restoration of all things in the new creation. The story passes directly through the cross of Christ and proceeds through the Church, the bride whom Jesus has raised up to shine the light

> **Without the grand story of the Bible, we may inadvertently communicate that healing is in the medical care itself and that sickness and health are not God's concern or in His control.**

of His Kingdom in the world. We need the solid reality of this story as a sure foundation for the mission of God through healthcare.

The period of healthcare missions: the late twentieth century through today

The pace of growth of mission hospitals quickened during the first half of the twentieth century but declined markedly during the second half. The colonial era was coming to a close, and newly independent nations were forming, especially after WWII in the middle of the century. The fruit of the first 150 years of evangelism and mission medical care included both churches and more advanced hospital care. Hospitals were becoming increasingly expensive and challenging for mission organizations to manage. Many hospitals were handed over to local church partners, and the new governments nationalized others. Churches and mission agencies alike were concerned that specialization was increasing the cost of care and diverting it from the poor. A change was needed, but what kind of change?

By the 1980s and 1990s, mission agencies were introducing a new model of community health, fashioned after the World Health Organization's (WHO) Primary Health Care (PHC) declaration in 1978 at Alma-Ata. Alma-Ata underscored "revolutionary principles—equity, social justice, and health for all; community participation; health promotion; appropriate use of resources; and intersectoral health."[160] WHO changed its focus from the management of specific diseases to primary healthcare. The flurry of

---

[160] Lawn, J.E., Rodhe, J., Rifkin, S., et al. *"Alma Ata 30 years on: Revolutionary, Relevant, and time to Revitalize,"* The Lancet 372, issue 9642 (September 13, 2008): 917-927. https://doi.org/10.1016/S0140-6736(08)61402-6

building hospitals that had characterized the first half of the century died down, replaced by shorter-term projects. Institution building gave way to time-limited community health and development efforts, e.g. malaria and tuberculosis projects. This second period of medical missions is frequently called "healthcare mission" in order to emphasize this new holistic approach to health. And yet the changes introduced through PHC began to move us away from evangelism and medical care—the two powerful purposes we encountered in the first period.

This significant shift was based on WHO's interaction with the World Council of Churches' Christian Medical Commission (CMC). In turn, the CMC was informed by consultations with mainline churches and missions at the German Institute for Medical Missions in Tubingen, Germany in 1964. The impetus for the change in direction was meant to challenge a narrow view of medical mission, seen as "primarily a means of proselytizing, or saving bodies to save souls."[161] This challenge to evangelism tore at the fabric of God's mission.

WHO's PHC movement was born partly from the work of concerned Christians who wanted to address foundational issues like the role and function of mission hospitals. But rather than return to a biblical understanding of healing (the bigger story of the Kingdom of God), the movement challenged the very notions on which the medical mission enterprise was built: evangelism and medical care. Unfortunately, there was little effort to return to the drawing board and ask how evangelism and medical care could be

---

[161] Bersagel B. M., 'The Christian Medical Commission and the World Health Organization', in Ellen L. Idler (ed.), *Religion as a Social Determinant of Public Health* (New York, 2014; online edn, Oxford Academic, 18 Sept. 2014), https://doi.org/10.1093/acprof:oso/9780199362202.003.0021

better aligned, making needed repairs to the worldview of the first century and a half of medical missions.

If the assumptions of the earlier period sometimes conveyed that healing is found *in* medical care, the new PHC assumptions tended to convey that healing is found *outside* of medical care—in the church and community. Many of the examples and models of community transformation given were led by Christians who sought to minister to the poor with dignity. In the atmosphere of academics, however, the spiritual roots of these efforts were downplayed by secular enthusiasts.

One such project is the good work of Drs. Raj and Mabelle Arole in India. Still a model today, the Jamkhed project has served 500,000 rural poor and marginalized in Maharashtra state in India over the last 45 years.[162] Dedicated Christian workers have developed creative approaches to community health, shaped by gospel thinking. The PHC movement fashioned under WHO and the Christian Medical Commission expressly wanted to avoid "saving bodies to save souls."[163] The work of God to bring about community transformation was seldom acknowledged.

The PHC movement challenged *not only* the focus of medical missions on evangelism *but even* the medical approach itself! David Jenkins, Head of Theology and Religious Studies at the University of Leeds wrote, "Christianity can be seen as mixed up with Western Imperialism, and medicine can be seen as a set of expensive technologies run by professionals who may be pursuing their own interests quite as much as, if not more than, promoting the health

---

[162] *CRHP Comprehensive Rural Health Project Jamkhed.* https://www.crhpindia.org/

[163] Bersagel, "The Christian Medical Commission and the World Health Organization," 7.

of communities and individuals within society."[164] Medical professionals were seen more as the problem than part of the solution. "To the Christian of today the ministry of healing is very often thought of in terms of *professional* service alone–perhaps even in a distant country–having very little connection with the life of the congregation."[165]

By the middle of the twentieth century, the mission of Christian hospitals, which had been shaped, if imperfectly, by the gospel, came under suspicion. Surveys had found that "the churches had concentrated their efforts on building and operating hospital and clinic-based curative services which had a limited impact on the problems in the community. They were, basically, repair facilities that did little if anything to remove the causes of sickness or to promote and maintain health."[166]

To address the issues facing medical missions, the Tubingen consultation emphasized that all healing is from God, so the church has a central role in the healing ministry. The focus became preventive care in the community. There is much good and right about that emphasis. The problem is that some PHC efforts stressed the community almost to the exclusion of care for the sick in hospitals. Paradoxically, returning healing ministry to the church[167] marginalized the historical emphasis on care for the sick in hospitals and clinics! Clinical care, in Jesus' name, was sidelined and sometimes

---

[164] McGilvray, J.C., *The Quest for Health and Wholeness* (Tubingen: German Institute for Medical Missions, 1981), ix.

[165] *The Healing Church: The Tubingen Consultation 1964, World Council of Churches, Geneva 1965* (World Council Studies 3, Published by Difam, German Institute for Medical Missions), 36/37. https://worldea.org/wp-content/uploads/2020/02/Tuebingen-I-1964english.pdf

[166] McGilvray, *The Quest for Health and Wholeness*, xv.

[167] *The Healing Church: The Tubingen Consultation 1964*, 34/35.

even stigmatized. And despite good intentions, the new PHC effort also tended to devalue evangelism. These influences have created new challenges for the healthcare mission enterprise today.

Assumptions during this period of healthcare mission

I must confess that the emphasis on primary healthcare over the past 50 years has greatly influenced my own career. I was a student in International Health under Dr. Carl Taylor, a leading originator of the work of the Christian Medical Commission of the World Council of Churches. He was a role model and an influential Christian statesman for community health. He understood the need for balancing primary, secondary, and tertiary medical care. I saw the value of the PHC approach through his eyes, but, over time, became aware of some of its limitations. Despite good intentions, the movement challenged, and sometimes even damaged, the historic roots of healthcare at the bedside.

Having spent my career as a clinician and an epidemiologist, I've seen the need for a combined approach (prevention and treatment) numerous times. Women need birthing care as close as feasible to their homes in Nepal since they are often separated from hospitals by mountain ranges. And yet there must be a system to identify high-risk women and refer them to hospitals. Similar arguments are easily made for TB, motor vehicle accidents, and a host of other conditions. Prevention and treatment are complementary, not in competition. Healthcare must be both-and, not either-or! To encompass both, our vision for healthcare must be informed by God's design for creation and redemption. Any other story is inadequate, and prone to error and failure.

The medical mission enterprise has grown up under the cultural influence of our modern secular-sacred divide, driven by the twin purposes of healthcare (often based on secular training) and gospel ministry (sometimes seemingly unconcerned about this world). The story of the gospel must unify these purposes under the mission of God. Rather than returning to a ministry to the sick which stretches back to the days of Jesus, however, the founders of the PHC movement moved away from historic Christianity. The outward form of Christianity was kept but the heart of the gospel was often lost. This is like throwing the baby out with the bathwater!

> **God's design for *both* creation *and* redemption must form our vision for healthcare.**

The very role and place of medical missions was called into question during this recent move to PHC and the community. Tubingen's emphasis was a "fundamental challenge to what was traditionally understood as the twofold task of medical missions: meeting physical needs and preaching the Gospel."[168] *Rather than addressing the issues of sustainability and purpose of mission hospitals, the movement had proposed a redefinition of mission!* The role of missionary medicine came under threat. And while there remain fine examples of healthcare mission today, my concern is that we must move toward, not away from, our biblical foundations. If we are able to do that we will find, I hope, that medical and healthcare emphases can (and should) be quite integrated.

---

[168] Bersagel, "The Christian Medical Commission and the World Health Organization," 2.

The PHC movement from Tubingen emphasized the Kingdom of God, community, prevention, and the need for social justice. This was helpful since treating the sick in hospitals without thinking of the suffering at the community level is shortsighted. But the worldview behind the new model, while seemingly spiritual, did not embrace the gospel story the way that Jesus did. Jesus' healing ministry was welcomed, but not His emphasis on repentance, faith, and the forgiveness of sin. Instead, health was described as an "involvement with Jesus in the victorious encounter of the Kingdom of God with the powers of evil."[169] While it is vital to combat evil, salvation from sin is the heart of Jesus' ministry. While the movement used the term "Kingdom of God," it was not the same "Kingdom of God" that Jesus proclaimed.

The PHC movement, perhaps with a sincere attempt to correct the limitations of the first period of medical missions, promoted a different gospel. The promoters used spiritual language to discuss important issues like justice and *shalom* but were less focused on (at times perhaps indifferent to) the need for repentance and forgiveness. Without the work of Jesus Christ on the cross, there is no healing and no power to change people.

Many voices today promote a gospel of the Kingdom that focuses on good works but minimizes the need for repentance from sin and faith in Christ's work on the cross for sinners. Pastor Greg Gilbert writes:

> *Again and again, in book after book, we see descriptions of the gospel that end up relegating the cross to a secondary position. In its place are declarations that the heart of the gospel*

---

[169] *The Healing Church: The Tubingen Consultation 1964*, 35/36.

is that God is remaking the world or that He has promised a Kingdom that will set everything right, or that He is calling us to join Him in transforming culture. Whatever the specifics, the result is that over and over again, the death of Jesus in the place of sinners is assumed, marginalized, or even (sometimes deliberately) ignored.[170]

It is true that God is remaking the world and establishing His Kingdom; to join Him, our first concern must be to repent and believe.[171]

What story is this second period of healthcare missions communicating?

The PHC emphasis over the past 50 years has resulted in a proliferation of agencies and organizations to address health needs at the societal level. This is a good thing. To emphasize the new focus on health rather than disease, many mission agencies began using the term "healthcare missions" instead of "medical missions." This communicates that we want to see a ministry to the whole person and the whole community. This is a good change and aligns with what we have learned about God's mission. Preventive care and restorative care must be done together in missional healthcare. The gospel story weaves them together!

We must avoid a false dichotomy between clinical care and community care. This is a both-and situation, not either-or. In the same way, we must avoid a dichotomy between spiritual and physical ministry. This, too, is a both-and situation, not either-or.

---

[170] Gilbert, G., *What is the Gospel?* (Wheaton: Crossway Books, 2010), 35.

[171] For one of many examples, see Jesus' first announcement of the Kingdom of God in Mark 1:15

Healing is not found inside *or* outside of medical care. Healing is a gift of God, not found in the medical profession, the church, or the community. Only the true story of the Bible will keep us balanced, integrating medical care with church and community care. It allows us to integrate ministry to the body with ministry to the soul.

I love the emphasis of the PHC movement on the church. I love the move toward the community, aiming to prevent illness rather than only treat it. I love the emphasis on *shalom* and on God's concern with the whole of life. The danger is that the story has sometimes become what *we* can do as Christians to transform the world. I have seen community-based efforts that minimize the seriousness of our sin problem. We risk promoting a different gospel if we communicate (even inadvertently) that *we* will build the Kingdom rather than let Christ work through us. (We also put a big burden on ourselves. It is a recipe for burnout!)

Disease care at the bedside and preventive efforts in the community both contribute to human flourishing. The mission of God must involve both! Each has a part in God's mission: He makes disciples who change the world by following Jesus. That mission encompasses physical health but is wider than health. *Shalom* includes all God intended in creation for human flourishing (and more!). Whether in the clinic or community, that *shalom* flows out of people who have repented of sin and trust in Christ; it is not independent of Him.

The global impact for Christ would be multiplied if we could create better synergy between those who do individual care, community work, and non-health ministries, especially those that reach people for Christ and build them up. The synergy we need must be founded on Scripture. This kind of synergy enables us to plan our healthcare activities without dissonance between physical and spiritual ministries. Are we as passionate about making disciples as much as we are about delivering quality medical care? Are we eager to connect with churches and the community in order to multiply our efforts? A big picture of God's work in the world enables this synergy.

We can start small. A doctor couple in Ethiopia was working in a remote clinic. They asked permission to visit the homes of patients they had seen in the clinic. This created a challenge for the schedule, but the clinic leader permitted a trial. They followed up with patients in their homes and taught the Bible through oral storytelling. While visiting one particular child for follow-up, they gained quite an audience from the surrounding houses during the Bible story. They were welcomed back to that home, where some women came to faith. Catching their vision, the clinic leader allowed clinic staff to participate in the experiment; soon they caught a vision and continued the ministry. The work grew through evangelism (the village people and friends), discipleship (the healthcare workers), and church planting (the group that grew up and continued to meet and worship). In the end, God received the glory, and the people in the community were blessed.

This new emphasis on PHC has the potential to demonstrate to churches how the Lord can use healthcare to reach communities. It can communicate the beauty of partnership. It can model whole-person ministry, especially as local believers catch a vision for the mission of God. Partnering with one another (especially clinical and community health workers) will demonstrate the gospel's power rather than simply our programs' strengths. Working with other non-health ministries, such as church planting and theological education, enables us to honor the King and participate in the Kingdom He is building. It can change cultures.

As we enter the next century of healthcare missions, may the Lord enable us to humbly shape it according to the bigger story of God's work in transforming the nations.

Questions for reflection:

How would you sum up the difference between the first and second periods of medical and healthcare missions to your students in healthcare?

What are the advantages and disadvantages of separating evangelism and healthcare?

I have argued that the Kingdom of God, biblically understood, is key to understanding God's mission in the world, and yet it is frequently misrepresented. How do you react?

PART IV

Serving with God's Purpose

CHAPTER 11

Leadership in Healthcare Mission

I was asked to help evaluate whether we should close one of our hospitals in crisis. The hospital was founded on the twin purposes of surgery and evangelism, but decades later, a conflict arose. The head surgeon wanted to expand the evangelistic impact by adding more surgical capacity. The head nurse knew that meant burning out nurses already working at capacity. The surgeon felt that the work should be driven by his agenda, in line with the hospital's founding. The nurse asked, "Should work alone drive the agenda, with no consideration for the well-being of staff?" Neither was willing to step back and consider how to care for *both* patients *and* staff.

In frustration, the nurse did something practical and effective, at least in the short run. To block the doctor's expansion plans, she hid the extra needed hospital beds in an unused storage room where they could not be found. In the long run, however, without common ground, leadership remained a power struggle.

It was not just the foreign missionary staff that could not find common ground. I discovered the national staff, too, was planning to strike. They were frustrated that their views on the ministry were never considered. With all these conflicts, the hospital was losing its gospel witness. Yet women and children had nowhere else to go for healthcare. I wrestled with the question of closure, asking myself, "What is the real problem here?" I concluded that the problem was not overwork or the pressing needs. The real problem was the lack of leadership. Eventually, the Lord did provide an African physician as the new hospital director, who led in such a way that everyone was heard; the hospital culture and ministry began to reflect the love of Christ.

Leadership is ministry. Without leadership, a Christian healthcare ministry can remain stuck in unhealthy patterns. Godly leaders are essential to tackle current issues and shape the future. You may be a healthcare professional or a mission leader responsible for healthcare workers. Either way, godly leadership is essential for a healthy ministry.

Most of us in healthcare are comfortable in the fields we have trained in. I love general internal medicine and primary health care. I am also very comfortable with epidemiology, using a different set of tools to promote the health of communities. We tend to hold onto our culture, including our professional identity, when we begin working in a different culture and language. But comfort can also be limiting. As you adjust to a new culture and language, consider moving beyond the limits of your medical specialty. Trust God to also take you deeper into the waters of spiritual leadership.

I stepped into a leadership role after serving some years as a missionary physician and epidemiologist. Rather than direct care, I was asked to help other medical missionaries thrive. This stretched me because I was less comfortable with soft, fuzzy relationships than with secure clinical guidelines and case-control studies. Through the experience of leadership, I learned the importance of governance, systems thinking, and developing people. Without solid, godly leadership, good intentions can get sidetracked by conflict, loss of vision, and mission drift. The Lord began to show me the benefits of servant leadership.

You may recall that many mission hospitals were started in the twentieth century by medical doctors, often surgeons, who had the determination to get things done. These well-meaning doctors had a passion for both medical care and evangelism. And while God used them for a time, many of these institutions were eventually handed over to the government or churches. Some of them lost their original mission in the transition, partly because of inadequate preparation of new leadership. A hospital may be managed well enough to keep things operational, but it eventually needs more than day-to-day management. It takes godly leadership and visionary governance to tune the ministry over time to the melody of the Kingdom of God.

A survey of forty-three church hospitals in Africa and Asia identified criteria for sustainability. The top three items specified were: 1) mission vision, 2) visionary governance, and 3) dynamic leadership.[172] The ministry of leadership was thought to be even more important than quality, staffing, and finances! The gospel is

---

[172] Asante, R.K.O., *Sustainability of Church Hospitals in Developing Countries* (World Council of Churches, 1998), 71.

the ultimate source of these leadership gifts. Money, for example, is not the source of sustainability. The Apostle Paul speaks of the gospel as that "which has come to you, just as in all the world it is constantly bearing fruit and increasing." (Col 1:6).

Famed management consultant Peter Drucker tells a story about good management and leadership:

> *Three stonecutters were asked what they were doing. The first replied, "I am making a living." The second kept on hammering while he said, "I am doing the best job of stonecutting in the entire country." The third one looked up with a visionary gleam in his eyes and said, "I am building a cathedral." The third man is, of course, the true manager [leader]. The first man knows what he wants to get out of the work and manages to do so. He is likely to give a fair day's work for a fair day's pay. But he is not a manager [leader] and will never be one. It is the second man who is the problem. Workmanship is essential. An organization demoralizes if it does not demand of its members the highest workmanship they are capable of. But there is always a danger that the true workman, the true professional, will believe that he is accomplishing something when, in effect, he is just polishing stones or collecting footnotes. Workmanship must be encouraged in the business enterprise. But it must always be related to the needs of the whole.[173]*

---

[173] Drucker, P.F., *Management Tasks, Responsibilities, Practices* (Harper Collins, 1973). See *ThEME – The Elements of management effectiveness.* (1973). https://www.nycp.com/elements/HA1/1345#:~:text=The%20first%20replied%2C%20'I%20am,of%20course%2C%20the%20true%20manager.

Good leaders are hard to find! Some of us are too reluctant. Others are too confident and become authoritarian commanders rather than shepherds, servants, and stewards of God's work. You will invariably be a leader in some capacity during your career in healthcare missions. What kind of leader will you be?

The task of leadership in healthcare ministry

A missionary colleague and biomedical engineer once described his conversation with the hospital engineers he was trying to train in India.

He said, "These electrical transformers need your attention for regular maintenance. You have not touched them for months!"

"It is better if we don't interfere with them, boss," they replied.

"But if you don't maintain them, they will start to buzz and vibrate, and the power may surge unexpectedly. The electric poles may come down, and we could lose power to the whole hospital," he exclaimed.

The hospital engineers responded, "Ah, Sir, that's the trouble. If we maintain them all the time, no one will appreciate our work!"

What is the task of leadership about? According to these engineers, leadership is about showing how important *we* are. But that's not the case. Christian author Henry Blackaby says, "Spiritual leadership is about moving people onto God's agenda."[174] Leadership is about moving beyond today to a vision of the future. We need managers to make organizations and programs stable and efficient. Even more desperately, we need leaders who will spend time with God and others, hear the pain of brokenhearted people, and shape

---

[174] Blackaby, H. and Blackaby, R., *Spiritual Leadership* (Nashville: Broadman and Holman, 2001), 20.

the program or institution to advance the cause of Christ, not ourselves. Leadership keeps healthcare ministry aligned with God's agenda by bringing people together around purpose.

The key is "for spiritual leaders to understand God's will for them and their organizations."[175] It does not mean becoming an expert in finances, strategic planning, or developing systems. These things are necessary, but others on leadership teams may do them better. If you are a leader, the *one* thing you cannot delegate is the vision of the ministry and its connection with God's mission. Identifying, embracing, and communicating the mission's purpose and direction may be a leader's most important task.

We have discovered that cultural or worldview assumptions can derail healthcare from the mission of God. When science dominates our thinking, and God's revelation is compartmentalized, the work of the Kingdom will be distorted. When medical professionals and scientists first seek His Kingdom and righteousness, science and medicine will find their proper places. As Westerners, I fear we have too often "lost the story" of redemption. Instead, we have a story about bodily health (too earthly-minded) or spiritual salvation (too heavenly-minded). The work of Jesus is about integrating them under Heaven's direction.

Leadership means partnership, not isolation. A Kingdom-oriented healthcare leader may ask, "How can we as healthcare disciples help churches reach out to communities where Christ is least known? How can we work together?" A Kingdom-oriented mission leader, although not medical, may ask, "How might we use healthcare ministry as part of our strategy to reach suffering communities with the gospel?" Leadership in healthcare mission is not

---

[175] Ibid., 23.

leadership in church planting per se. But to advance the Kingdom, both types of leaders must walk hand-in-hand to enrich each other's ministries. Healthcare can play a vital role in alleviating suffering and helping plant healthy churches to make a long-term impact on the community.

For example, the hospital could find ways to be a resource or training ground for church volunteers who want to serve in the community. The church could help the hospital by supporting local Christian healthcare workers (professionals) or workers in training. It might find other practical ways to help those who want to give their lives for the Lord's service. Christian author Amy Sherman describes this mindset as "vocational stewardship for the common good."[176] Trinity Dental Clinic in Liberia has been training dental assistants who will work with churches to serve communities without dental care. Trinity leaders partnered with an association of churches to help define the ministry and select and deploy these new dental assistants. Not only will they provide much-needed primary dental care in selected villages, but these village churches will also help them minister to the whole person. This kind of partnership can only come about as healthcare leaders build relationships of trust with others.

> **If you are a leader, the *one* thing you cannot delegate is the vision of the ministry and its connection with God's mission.**

---

[176] Sherman, A.L., *Kingdom Calling – Vocational Stewardship for the Common Good* (Downers Grove: IV Press, 2011), 99.

A missionary physician and his wife have served in a hospital in rural South Africa for decades. He is no longer needed in patient care or hospital leadership but works with the Christian Medical Fellowship in South Africa to mentor younger doctors and medical professionals. He has begun to accompany some younger ones to hospitals in Zambia, Zimbabwe, and the Island nations. He is working with churches to help them gain a vision for God's mission beyond South Africa. He would not consider himself a church planter but truly has the heart of one. We are not all church planters, but we can have a vision for planting churches—and communicate this through our lives.

Healthcare leaders can help national Christian staff find innovative ways to care for marginalized communities, using what they have learned as disciples in the hospital or health program. This could mean intentionally investing in those who want to serve communities in need through training and deploying them. It would take sacrifice for the institution to contribute personnel or finances to a community health project. It would also be a sacrifice for the individual, who might take little or no pay. Outreaches to serve people who cannot pay back can be costly to those who serve.

Too often, churches have seen hospitals as a means of income rather than an investment in the community. Godly, Kingdom-oriented leadership can save us from this myopic vision. The hospital or healthcare ministry does not exist for itself, but neither does the church! One way to foster healthy partnerships with local churches is to create hospital governing boards that represent not only patient interests but community interests as well. Local believers and churches can provide a much-needed role on such boards. Our high calling together is to join with Christ to shape the culture of the world and enable others to flourish under God by making disciples. In healthcare that means making a difference inside the institution or organization that we are part of, with a view towards justice and righteousness.

The how of leadership in healthcare

In Chapter Two, Bruce had to decide if he was willing to face up to his own vulnerability as a leader of the medical staff. Like Bruce, I began my mission career thinking about my technical performance, unaware of my fear of failure. Our discipleship journey is not as much about having flawless skills as our willingness to be vulnerable and grow in Christlikeness. This kind of openness also builds leaders!

Christian anthropologist Sherwood Lingenfelter has written a helpful guide to forging ministry in the crucible of crisis, *Leadership in the Way of the Cross*. His words are pertinent: "This process begins with self-discovery–disclosing default habits, fears, and hungers– followed by trusting the Holy Spirit to work God's transformation within us, and then engaging in the hard work of mobilizing his body, the people of God, so that every part is doing his work."[177]

Becoming a good leader is more than just getting good information and knowledge. It means being the person God is making us to be. Nothing compares to learning on the job. The crucible of cross-cultural healthcare is one of the best places to develop leadership skills, especially if one can find some trusted mentors. One of my mentors, Dr. Andrew Ng, would say, "It's like getting a Ph.D. in

---

[177] Lingenfelter, S.G., *Leadership in the Way of the Cross – Forging Ministry from the Crucible of Crisis* (Eugene, OR: Cascade Books, 2018), 7.

leadership!" Godly leadership and discipleship are intimately connected, and both are learned on the job!

As a Christian healthcare worker, I have been learning to listen to my patients. I used to listen to the description of medical issues so I could find a solution. Now, I'm also listening to their spiritual needs, even as they describe their health concerns. I've found that careful listening to patients and staff opens opportunities to hear the needs of families and communities. The same listening skills are essential to leadership. I will not be able to meet all the needs of patients or staff, but leadership allows us to move our team onto God's agenda, God's mission. Learning to listen to others is crucial to making disciples *and* good healthcare. Only the Holy Spirit can mold our character so that we can both listen and humbly assert authority.

In a survey of medical missionaries, medical missionary and coach Jim Ritchie identified leadership and followership as top priorities. "Too often those who are in leadership are domineering, and those who are younger are resistant to a follower's role."[178] Leading like Jesus will mean listening to those who serve under us as well as those to whom we report. Leaders will be shepherds, servants, and stewards of the ones they are accountable to.[179] Leaders will disciple others but also be disciples.

Missiologist Andrew Walls reminds us that the missionary movement was designed for one-way traffic, for sending, for giving. Now is the time to find ways "better fitted for two-way traffic, for fellowship, for sharing, for receiving."[180] Many hospitals planted

---

[178] Jim Ritchie, personal communication, November 11, 2022.

[179] Bremner, D., *Images of Leadership: Biblical Portraits of Godly Leaders* (Oasis International, 2021).

[180] Walls, *The Missionary Movement in Christian History*, 260.

as mission hospitals now serve communities with better health and access to care. Sometimes churches have also been planted. Important questions must be answered about the direction for the future. Should we continue with the healthcare ministry? Do we close it? Or is God leading us to a particular health focus, such as women's health or people with disabilities? Is He leading us to focus on a particular poor community or segment of society? These are not just medical questions. Leadership means tackling them in trusting relationships with local churches and ministry partners.

In my experience as a Western missionary, it takes at least five years of service in another country to settle in, learn a new language and culture, establish your home (and family, if married), and learn the medical ropes. But as you develop capacity, look for opportunities to grow as a leader. Perhaps start with a small project or department, but don't be afraid to look beyond the daily routine and dream–with others–as to what God might do.

Western professionals often make complex and costly decisions to be able to serve long-term. In addition, our Western family systems are often more fragile, so it takes time to work through our own dysfunctions to have healthy relationships. There has been a clear trend for shorter terms of service even for "long-term" medical missionaries from the West. As non-Western professional brothers and sisters increasingly serve, leadership teams will become more multicultural.

At the same time, there has been wonderful growth of Christian healthcare workers globally. The International Christian Medical and Dental Association strengthens the hand of Christian medical professionals across chapters in more than 100 nations. Doctors, nurses, and health professionals from many of these nations are engaging in ministry to the poor both in their own countries and abroad. This shift towards multicultural teams will allow the giving and receiving of Walls' "two-way traffic of fellowship, sharing and receiving."

Meeting the challenge of the suffering of this world, especially among communities with limited resources, will take creative new initiatives. Rather than copy the world's methods, Christians who understand the cultural mandate and its connection to salvation have the perspective and wisdom to face global health challenges. It will take us as healthcare professionals outside of our comfort zones. It will take multicultural leadership, not just teamwork. We can trust the Holy Spirit to guide us since the work is important to God.

I have seen many emerging healthcare leaders and their dedication to the Lord. I have had the privilege of teaching a Christian Global Health in Perspective course for global ICMDA medical professionals. The student feedback from this course has been very encouraging. According to one of them, an academic dentist from Singapore, they are catching a vision for "the beautiful design of God's plan." An Indonesian brother commented, "The test of a society is the well-being of the least." A doctor serving in rural Thailand wants to share the "biblical metanarrative" of creation, Fall, and redemption with his fellow Thai students in public health.[181]

So how is healthcare leadership most effective? How do we serve the Lord as leaders in our hospitals and missions? We tackle some of the causes of poor health at the bedside but also in the community. As medical folks, we have the privilege of being received

---

[181] These are comments from a debrief after one of our 12-week courses online: *Christian Global Health in Perspective* (https://www.cghiperspective.com/) produced by Health for All Nations (https://www.healthforallnations.com/).

into the homes of people we have served–the mother whose child the midwife delivered or the older adult whom we were able to help with some small act of kindness. Leadership sees every encounter with patients as an opportunity to develop trust, which can open doors. Leaders will enable their programs and institutions to make disciples to strengthen their own ministry as well as extend the reach of ministries into local communities.

Is God calling you to leadership?

Like many, you may be saying, "Who, me? A leader?" You may think yourself too busy, unqualified, or not spiritually ready. I would encourage you to consider leadership as a means of changing the future, not just managing the present. Without vision, people perish, and without leadership, there is no advancement of God's vision for human flourishing through Christ.

In *Ideas Have Consequences*, Richard Weaver warns us of the extinction of the idea of mission: "Men no longer feel it laid upon them to translate the potential into the actual; there are no goals of labor like those of the cathedral-builders."[182] To spend one's life to relieve a little bit of the tremendous suffering of the world and to make disciples in the process that will extend and broaden that impact for time and eternity–that is a cathedral worth building.

We need leaders who have not just a vision of expediency but who value the people who do the work. Let's use the projects to develop the people, not the other way around. Above all, our healthcare ministries need wisdom. Since you, as Christ's child,

---

[182] Weaver, R.M., *Ideas Have Consequences* (University of Chicago, 1948), 116.

have access to all His wisdom (see James 1), consider what Christ may be calling you to accomplish.

During our time in Ethiopia, I received an urgent message for our church leader from his son, who was studying in England. To deliver it by hand (before the day of email), I took my family and a young man in my health discipleship group and drove up the 4,000-foot escarpment to his home. I mentioned earlier that the church leaders were not consulted when the mission first placed us in our location, and this particular church leader felt the "rift between church and mission" quite acutely. Upon our arrival, he gave us the cold shoulder, making us wait a considerable time before receiving us, very unlike traditional Ethiopian culture. Years later, long after I had forgotten about this young man, I met him again at a mission gathering. He had become a mature leader in the denomination, responsible for all mission outreaches. Somehow this incident had made a deep impression on him. He said, "I was so embarrassed by the treatment you received from my own people, but you were able to take it without offense." The Holy Spirit was building into his life without my knowledge. He is leaving a legacy; he is a cathedral builder. I could see that God had arranged these things beforehand for His purposes. Small things can make a big difference even if they only touch one person.

Leadership means developing relationships of trust with national colleagues as well as churches and others passionate about the mission of God. It means tackling impossible questions with the wisdom of the Spirit of God found in trusted partnerships. My former SIM Director, Bruce Johnson, said, "Put community before committee." This will result not just in more efficient and effective operations but in more God-glorifying and gospel-loving disciples.

A biblically informed worldview will help us and our national colleagues address the cultural issues that challenge us. Putting healthcare ministry on a solid, long-term foundation means that every culture needs to be shaped by the gospel narrative. We want to build our healthcare missions not on the models of the past or even on the fashions of the present but with a gospel-inspired, God-given vision for the future. God's Kingdom is not just about healthy bodies for this life but about lives changed for eternity through repentance and faith in Christ.

In our important work in healthcare, we get to touch the lives of human beings, the most fantastic creation of God, and help them find wholeness. This is a lifetime journey. That journey will have different seasons, but God may ask you to build on your early experiences to extend His work through the ministry of leadership. Embrace that season when God calls you to follow Him and then lead others in the mission of God.

Questions for reflection:

Why is leadership so important, and why does it sometimes give us so much trouble?

Do you identify more with the second or third stonecutter? Do you have so much passion for work that you lose the bigger picture?

What difference could you make by taking on a leadership role that would allow you to better "own" the mission and its direction?

Where are you in the process of self-discovery of "default habits, fears and hungers"?

CHAPTER 12

Following Christ's Call in Healthcare

In 1993 SIM's coordinator for community service ministries, Don Stilwell, initiated a consultation on health and development ministries in Nairobi. Medical missions had been an important part of SIM for 100 years, and he was responsible for ensuring ongoing impact. Medical missionaries and local African church partners were invited to the consultation. The Africans were encouraged to speak about ways SIM people sometimes hinder good partnerships.

"Now that we are becoming partners, please share your secret manual with us," insisted our African brothers and sisters.

Dismayed, Don asked them, "Why would you think SIM has a secret manual? There is no such thing."

"But we know there is a secret manual, and we all agree," they persisted.

When SIM mission leaders asked, "Why?" they responded: "Because every new generation of SIM medical missionaries *keeps making the same mistakes!*"

Don later wrote, "The behaviors listed revealed 'an unfortunate level of unworthy attitudes and behaviors on the part of some of our missionaries.'"[183] Although we (SIM) were proud of our medical mission efforts, we had to be ready for the discovery of some of our cultural blind spots.

"The Secret Manual"
Uncovered in Nairobi at the Community Services Ministry Consultation

When the time came for the discussion groups to report, the church partner participants listed a number of behaviors of SIM missionaries which they considered a hindrance to good church/mission partnerships. The following is the list they presented, roughly in order of significance:

- *Superior attitude*
- *Lack of openness*
- *Lack of respect for culture*
- *Favoritism*
- *No recognition of nationals (avoiding African doctors in hospital)*
- *No financial disclosure*
- *Hiding experiences*

---

[183] Stilwell, D., "Community Services Ministry Consultation Report and Recommendations to International Council" in *SIM Ministries Manual*, SIM Archives, Charlotte, NC. 1993

- *Use of old manual*
- *Pushiness*
- *Divide and rule system*
- *Carryover culture*
- *Being higher paid*
- *Not calling people in low work positions by name*

In addition, one African participant, in his plenary presentation, mentioned:

- *Bad missionary attitudes (not corresponding to sacrifices made)*
- *Colonialist attitudes*
- *Master-servant relationships*
- *Hands in pockets while worshiping or praying*
- *Not taking time to greet, befriend, sleep, and eat with partners*
- *Not sharing one's own time, life, family*
- *Selling used articles that might be given*
- *Not giving in keeping with their level of income*
- *Not listening (except to favorites and friends)*

Superior attitude? Lack of openness? Lack of respect for culture? These are the exact opposite of why most of us are involved in healthcare among the poor. How could we possibly get it so wrong? How could we be so blind?

Things are not always what they should be, and sometimes that's because of our own blindness. The good news is that we have faithful brothers and sisters around the world to help us. These attitudes and behaviors tell us something about our love for efficiency and our tendency to manage our world. Even well-intentioned missionaries are sometimes shaped more by culture than by Christ.

This book has shown that the cultural perceptions of Christian health workers shape our understanding of the mission task. False assumptions distort our expectations and our worldviews. A distorted understanding of God's purpose in the world undermines our well-meaning efforts. Richard Lints tells us that "Adults who are not driven by a theological vision will be driven by a vision of expediency."[184] Scripture re-orients us towards God-directed purpose and mission.

William Osler is known as the father of modern medicine and helped create the medical education system at Johns Hopkins. He was a man of faith, especially faith in humanity and the medical profession.[185] His *Counsels and Ideals* reflect this modern worldview. He told his students, "Every one of you will have to face the ordeal of every student in this generation who sooner or later tries to mix the waters of science with the oil of faith. You can have a good deal of both *if you only keep them separate*."[186] He suggested that physicians maintain objectivity by focusing on medicine as something apart from faith.[187] This perspective keeps God at a distance from our healthcare work.

How prone we are to be charmed by the world. Christopher Wright points out that Western Christianity has been infected with

---

[184] Lints, *The Fabric of Theology*, 335.

[185] Osler, W. (1910). THE FAITH THAT HEALS. *BMJ*, 1(2581), 1470–1472. https://doi.org/10.1136/bmj.1.2581.1470

[186] Osler, W., *Counsels and Ideals* (London: Oxford University Press, 1921), 248. [Italics mine.]

[187] Ibid., 248.

cultural idolatry.[188] We want a certain amount of faith for respectability, but not enough to challenge and change us. Healthcare and gospel ministries can each take on a life of their own. The only remedy for us is to wholeheartedly embrace the message of the gospel in every aspect of life and work.

Jesus has purchased salvation for sinners on the cross. The fruit of that purchase, however, spans time and space, encompassing all of history. Sauer says, "The history of the ages is the history of mankind, and the history of mankind is the history–of God."[189] The effect of Christ's purchase is a coherent story of God's work in history. This gospel story shows why God's purpose includes bodily healing. God uses suffering, death, and healing as a theatre to communicate our need and his provision for our need. This story helps make sense of suffering and points us all to the grace of God. It should help us make sense of our journey in Christian healthcare ministry.

Let's wrap up, review what we have covered, and chart the next steps.

Where have we come from?

I began this book by describing some of my own challenges as I started my mission career in Ethiopia. It was a bumpy ride. I discovered that, despite all my training, I was not thriving. As a growing disciple, I was beginning to discover how the role of a doctor fits into God's story. Chapter Two highlighted the challenges

---

[188] Wright, C. J. H., "An Upside-Down world," *ChristianityToday.com*, January 18, 2007, 2, https://www.christianitytoday.com/ct/2007/january/30.42.html?utm_medium=widgetsocial

[189] Sauer, *The Dawn of World Redemption*, 15.

of our fictional but realistic missionary nurses and doctors. Some found healing and lasting joy in their journey; others did not. **Our ministry will not thrive unless we ourselves are growing as disciples of Christ.**

Jeremiah speaks of the priests who healed God's people superficially, crying "peace, peace" when there was no peace.[190] Man-made remedies are superficial. Wounded healers need healing. God provides the deep healing that we need through Scripture. Our healing includes an appreciation and acceptance of how we fit into the mission of God.

Christian healthcare ministry cares for others and helps them discover the duty and delight of fulfilling the cultural mandate. We learned in Chapter Three that God created the entire human race for a purpose. Under His Lordship, men and women were given the mandate to bring out the potential of the whole created world. This meant not only cultivating the garden and caring for animals but also enabling other human beings to flourish. This "cultural mandate" is God's design. Our responsibility as men and women on earth is to shape culture toward righteousness—God's perfect will for humankind and the world. Healthcare ministry expresses God's purpose by joining with God to bring about wholeness and *shalom*.

Christians in healthcare ministry will not focus on disease and brokenness without addressing sin, the root cause of our brokenness. Sin (Chapter Four) distorted God's purpose and led to brokenness in place of God's *shalom*. Our separation from God is the root cause of our disintegration. Because of sin, things became

---

[190] Jeremiah 6:14

"not the way they were supposed to be."[191] Moral decay brought physical decay. Suffering, disease, and death reflect the spiritual death we have chosen. Our pain is not just biological but points us to God and His intention to make us whole. Healthcare ministry allows us to enter into the suffering of others and say that bodily brokenness is not the whole story.

The message of salvation in Christ enables patients and communities to find meaning in suffering within the bigger story of God's Kingdom. Salvation (Chapter Five) restores the brokenness of creation because Christ has atoned for sin through His work on the cross. Resurrection points us to a renewed creation, fulfilling and surpassing the original. Since Christ is the true integration of all things, we can only find the wholeness God intended in Him. Bodily healing is not wholeness by itself but points us to God and the bigger story of salvation. *Shalom* is only possible in Christ.

The gospel is both spoken and seen through Christian healthcare ministry, but there is a special priority to spoken words. *Shalom* depends on words of faith which point us to the King. In a thought experiment, we imagined that Jesus healed every disease in the district of Capernaum and concluded that bodily healing alone was not enough. While Jesus loved to show compassion, He warned the crowds against following Him only to satisfy physical needs. We also tried to imagine what would have happened if Jesus had not physically healed people. We discovered that Christ's salvation changes us anyway, body and soul. We are healed from the inside out. Entering into the Kingdom of God through Jesus transforms communities and brings about holistic change which

---

[191] Plantinga, *Not the Way It's Supposed to Be*, 7-27.

we call *shalom*. Repentance and faith are the wellspring of shalom (Chapter Six).

Chapters Three to Six connect the themes of the gospel to healthcare. Any story needs a framework, a supporting structure on which it is built. The story of the gospel can be framed in three acts: creation, Fall, and salvation: a cosmic story of history seen from God's perspective. Healthcare ministry fits in the framework of the gospel story; it is not a separate story.

Having examined the framework for healthcare ministry, we considered the nature of ministry, with a history of ministries of compassion through the church. Then we turned to the nature of mission, including the last two hundred years of medical (now healthcare) mission. Aligning ministry and mission means partnering with the church in making disciples.

The calling of Jesus into healthcare ministry means being and making disciples (Chapter Seven). Jesus commanded this core activity in the Great Commission: "Go, make disciples of all nations." The gospel is the power of God to make disciples of individuals and nations. Disciples are not meant to lead private, heavenly-minded lives but instead live with their feet on the ground, engaged with the problems of the world, like Jesus. Disciples can enter into the suffering of others and join Him as He heals the brokenhearted and preaches good news to them. God uses them to shape the culture of all the peoples of the world for his glory.

In the last analysis, making disciples multiplies our impact. Our lives can make a certain amount of impact through medicine. But let us be defined by *how* we go about our medical work, loving others broken in body and spirit. Defining success as making disciples can help us set healthy boundaries and find greater satisfaction in our daily lives. A Christian calling to healthcare ministry is beautiful as we follow the steps of our Savior.

Partnering with churches and other Christians in disciple-making is God's means of shaping the cultures of the world according to His Kingdom. Centuries of compassionate care by churches helped us see the power of healthcare to change lives and shape culture. In Chapter Eight, we saw that the gospel motivated believers to move beyond their churches to serve the neglected. Hospitals set up for this purpose were a distinctly Christian signature of the gospel. Christian ministries to the poor over the centuries have shaped cultures and allowed many to come to know the Savior. Today, creative partnering with churches continues this legacy and allows us to have great impact for Christ.

Nurturing a passion for the mission of God in the world must be an important component of making disciples in healthcare. We focused on the bigger picture, the mission of God in Chapter Nine. It goes beyond healthcare ministries! Disciples who love the Lord will also embrace the mission of the church to bring the world under the Lordship of Christ. This "building of the Kingdom" is God's work, which God's people get to participate in through a variety of ministries. These disciples will grow to love God's church and other ministries and agencies involved in the mission of God.

Healthcare mission efforts today that are not motivated by the whole story of the Bible may find themselves driven to error, excess, and failure. Two hundred years of Protestant medical mission efforts provide inspiring examples of sacrificial service. They also caution us against defining medical mission as two separate categories, salvation of the soul (evangelism) and "salvation" of the body (medical care). Historian Mark Noll says, "Just as the past can deliver us from the smallness of [our] vision, so it can also caution us from error, excess, and failure."[192] The history of medical (now healthcare) missions underscores how false assumptions about medicine and the gospel can drive us towards either of these extremes (evangelism *or* healthcare). The biblical story of the mission of God gives a unified picture of the whole work of God in restoring creation as well as our place in that process (Chapter 10). It also keeps us from defining our work as "bringing in the Kingdom" but without emphasis on how one enters that Kingdom by repentance and faith.

Spiritual leadership for healthcare missions remains a key to advancing God's overall work of healing the creation and bringing the world under the Lordship of Christ. Christ continues to call us to God's missionary purpose through healthcare. We will face unique challenges which those who have gone before us have not. Where will we find the creativity needed for new approaches? Imagine what God can do as healthcare workers worldwide work together in this health-promoting, disciple-making movement! It will take godly leadership and relationships of trust to meet these challenges (Chapter 11).

What is next?

Where do we go from here? How do we put feet on what we have been learning?

Rather than just reading this book on your own, begin to discuss it with others. Share your thoughts with colleagues and friends. Mark down your notes and questions. How can we all work toward

---

[192] Noll, M.A., Hatch, N.O., Marsden, G.M., *The Search for Christian America* (Colorado Springs: Helmer and Howard, 1989), 146.

being disciples, making disciples, and making disciples across the cultures of the world?

Being a disciple takes more than intellectual prowess. Becoming a professional means graduating from training, but there is no graduation from being a disciple. Jesus is always conforming us to His image. Being a disciple means being a life-long learner of Jesus, learning how to live like Him in the world He has made. It can be a breathtaking journey, but it offers confidence and hope.

- Have you identified ways you have separated medical and spiritual agendas? Where can you find a place to share your journey with others?
- Are you paying attention to your inner life, not just outward success? Is there a prayer partner with whom you can share?
- Identify ways to define success (fruitfulness) more from the Bible than from culture. Do this in a community.
- Consider further training in history, the Bible, ethics, missiology, or leadership (not just in your medical specialization).
- Find creative ways of integrating healthcare and the communication of the gospel.
- Identify ways to address some of your own fears and anxiety in ministry and share these with a mentor.

Making disciples is the core ministry goal of both healthcare ministry and mission. I pray you will grow in your passion for making disciples, not as a program but as a lifestyle. Making disciples enables others to become life-long learners of Jesus. It is the secret to the growth of the Kingdom of God. It is the secret to changing cultures towards *shalom*.

- Can you identify false notions healthcare professionals have about disciple-making? Perhaps begin exploring this with a small group.
- Find ways of speaking not only about disease pathology but also about the meaning of illness to patients, especially ways of making God's purpose for humanity clearer (i.e., by sharing the gospel story).
- Develop creative ways to love patients well, not just as an individual practitioner but as a team. View every encounter with patients as an opportunity to address physical disease and human brokenness. Search for the brokenhearted with others on your team.
- Find some new ways to listen and learn from patients, community, and other believers. With others, address some of the roots of sickness, not just the manifestations.
- Develop your own coherent story of the place of healing in God's mission and challenge false assumptions both in the medical profession and in the church.
- As a disciple yourself, use the unique gifts and experiences God has given you to help others learn to integrate faith and practice.

Making disciples in another culture through healthcare lines up with God's purpose to enable human beings from every tribe, tongue, and nation to flourish. It means blessing those cultures and helping others conform to Christ's image rather than our own image. The blessing of *shalom* is a fruit of the resurrection of Jesus from the dead, coming to us by repentance and faith. What a joy to align our small lives with this big work of God to bless the nations!

- Consider your life in relation to what God is doing among the nations and orient your career – at least in part – to meet the needs of those who live in communities where Christ is least known and brokenness prevails. This may take you across the world or across your city.
- Take the time to learn what God is doing through others to proclaim the gospel through healthcare to unreached communities.
- Work with churches and mission leaders to integrate your medical ministry with other aspects of Great Commission work – where you are now and where Christ sends you. Address healthcare ministries and systems that are broken or built on false assumptions.
- Make disciples as healthcare teams, both in hospitals and clinics but also in communities.
- Develop relationships of trust with others who share a passion for healthcare among the poor and marginalized– especially on multicultural teams.
- Don't despise small beginnings and even failures as you seek to align healthcare ministry with the mission of God.

I began this book with a burden to speak with medical professionals serving Christ cross-culturally, both among the nations and domestically. I hope you have found ways in these pages to connect faith and practice at a deeper level. I pray that you will find a settled rest in meeting daily challenges with a wider perspective of God's purpose for you in discipling the nations.

Christopher Wright comments, "This God-centered refocusing of mission turns inside-out our obsession with mission plans, agendas, goals, strategies, and grand schemes. We ask, 'Where does God fit into the story of my life?' when the real question is, 'Where does my little life fit into the great story of God's mission?' We want to be driven by a purpose tailored for our individual lives when we should be seeing the purpose of all of life, including our own, wrapped up in the great mission of God for the whole of creation."[193]

I trust that you are ready to let God turn you inside out for His great glory and the healing of the nations!

---

[193] Wright, "An Upside-Down World," 4.

Appendices

APPENDIX A

A Liturgy for Medical Providers[194]

O Christ Our Healer,

There is no end to malady, sickness,
injury, and disease in this broken world,
so there is no end to the line of hurting
people who daily need my tending.

Therefore give me grace, O God,
that I might be generous with my kindness,
and that in this healing and care-taking vocation
my hands might become an extension of your
hands, and my service a conduit for your mercy.

---

[194] McKelvey, D., *Every Moment Holy* (Wheaton: Crossway Books, 2017), 44. Used with permission.

A Liturgy for Medical Providers

For it is often not an easy place to be –
    so near to suffering, to injury, to pain,
    to emergency and fear and confusion,
    and sometimes even to dying and
    death and grief –
but I believe it is exactly the sort of place
you would be, O Lord, amongst those
who hurt. So let my practice of medicine be
centered in an understanding of your heart.

Let me practice medicine
because you are a healing God
who feels compassion and extends mercy.
Let me practice medicine
because you are near to those who are in need,
to those who face grief and loss.
Let me practice medicine
as a willing servant of your redemption,
pushing back – by means of my vocation –
the effects of the fall.
Let my presence in this place lend a human face to your compassion.

Even when my schedule is crammed with
appointments, rounds, or duties, let me never
view my patients as mere tasks on a to-do-list.
Give me grace instead to be always –
even in our brief encounters –
attentive and responsive to the hearts
of human beings made in your image.

Let me extend kindness and mercy
even to those who are too angry, frightened,
bitter, or in pain to respond with anything but venom.
Let me especially love them, for they suffer –
even more than from physical ailment –
from a lack of understanding or experience
of your overwhelming grace and mercy and love.
Let their time with me be to them a taste
That might awaken a hopeful hunger in their hearts.

I can do none of these things on my own.
Apart from your grace, I have no grace to give.
So give me your grace in greater measure, O Lord.

Let me find also, in the midst of such constant need,
a rhythm of service and rest that will
enable my own soul to be tended and nourished –
that in the time I spend with patients
I will have a deeper repository of patience
and kindness to share with them.
Teach me how better to balance my duties
and my days, so that this work would not make me
absent from the lives of my family and friends and church.
Let me be well-woven into those communities
and relationships, enjoying ample time with them,
being available to them, and caring for their needs
even as I allow them to care for mine.
Let me never be so consumed by my vocation
that those closest to me
suffer negligence.

A Liturgy for Medical Providers

THE CLOSING SECTION MAY BE EXCERPTED FOR USE AS A SHORTER LITURGY

I would not just be a doctor or a nurse
or a medical provider, O God.
    I would be a minister of your healing
and compassion at work in your world.
    I would be a living witness of your love
expressed in a practical care of people.
    I would be your disciple in this place,
At this time, among this people.

So give grace, Lord Christ. Give me grace this day
and all days, that I might serve you well by loving
and serving others in this healing trade,
ever laboring in view of that day when
your Kingdom will be fully realized,
at the great mending of the world,
at the great ending of all ills.
Let me play a small part in that great work, today.

Amen

APPENDIX B

Recommended for Further Reading

* * *

The Gospel and the big picture of the Kingdom

Wright, Christopher J.H., *The Mission of God: Unlocking the Bible's Grand Narrative* **(Downers Grove: IVP Academic, 2006)**

Wright connects the story of redemption with the history of God's work in the whole world. He explores the global implications of themes such as Jubilee and the Exodus to help us see how God exercises his Kingship on behalf of the weak and oppressed. He wants us to see the ultimacy of evangelism, yet show us that mission without compassion and justice distorts the message of God. He argues that it is vital to see that every aspect of holistic, biblical mission (from evangelism to social concern) must be centered on the cross of Jesus.

Goheen, M.W. and Bartholomew, C.G., *The True Story of the Whole World – Finding Your Place in the Biblical Drama* (Michigan: Brazos Press, 2020)

This book tells the story of the Bible as a coherent drama "in order to subvert the powerful narrative that dominates our culture." The Bible tells the "real story" and thus provides a framework of meaning for all people and all times. We find meaning in brokenness and healing only within the framework of the real story.

Ashford, B.R. and Bartholomew, C.G., *The Doctrine of Creation* (Downers Grove: InterVarsity Press, 2020)

The Bible starts with creation and ends with a renewed creation (a new heaven and new earth). As a physician, I found that the emphasis in this book on creation helped me ground my worldview in the gospel without taking me out of this world. The authors say, "The Kingdom is about the recovery of God's purposes for His entire creation, through His Son." This book is like a basic science course for Christian healthcare ministry. It helped me understand that the line to be drawn is not between two aspects of creation, such as spirit and matter, but between God and His creation; that's where integration needs to be restored. That is basic science for doctors, nurses, and healthcare providers.

Kleinig, John W., *Wonderfully Made: A Protestant Theology of the Body* (Bellingham, WA: Lexham Press, 2021)

This book turns our attention to what living as human beings in the flesh means. The author calls it a "theological rhapsody on the body, a written reflection in praise of the human body… and praise of the triune God." With imagination and creativity, he shows us why the body matters to us, to one another, and to God.

Plantinga, C., *Not the Way It's Supposed to Be: A Breviary of Sin* (Grand Rapids: Eerdmans Publishing, 1995)

A very helpful, brief theology of sin. Our modern culture has obscured our understanding of sin. Plantinga sharpens our perception of sin and its effects, which ultimately make the world "not the way it's supposed to be." He helps us connect human suffering backward to the integrity of creation and forward to *shalom* and God's grace.

Geerhardus Vos, *The Kingdom of God* (Fontes Press, 2017 reprint of 1903 First edition)

Much confusion exists today over the nature of God's Kingdom. Vos was a professor of Biblical theology at Princeton a century ago but has produced a short and helpful look at the teachings of Jesus about the Kingdom of God. He shows the unity of Jesus' work with the Old Testament work of God. He paints a picture of the Kingdom as the renewal of the world, which has both "now" and "not yet" character. He shows how the Kingdom is not just an idea but an objective reality. This is an encouraging reminder of the significance of ministry to others who are suffering.

Christopher Watkin, *Thinking Through Creation: Genesis 1 and 2 as Tools of Cultural Critique* (P&R Publishing, 2017)

When God commanded Adam and Eve to fill the earth and subdue it, He mandated "that they go and make culture." Watkins delves into what creating culture implies, and concludes that God has created a world of meanings, but He invites us to create meaning together with Him, under His authority and guidance. Thus Adam named the animals, and we use language to shape ideas and create worlds. Are we as healthcare professionals shaped by the world's definition of disease and health? Or is our calling to shape that world, as Watkins urges us?

* * *

Healing and illness

Martin Lloyd-Jones, *Healing and the Scriptures* (Nashville: Thomas Nelson, 1988)

Lloyd-Jones was a beloved British pastor who left a promising medical career to enter the ministry. He wrote and spoke with authority on the intersection of faith and practice. He saw the dangers of professionalism in eclipsing the ministry to the whole person. While his writing is now half a century old, I suggest you read anything you can find by Dr. Martin Lloyd-Jones.

Jean-Claude Larchet, *The Theology of Illness* (St Vladimir's Seminary Press, 2002)

Larchet, a French Orthodox teacher, delves into the origins and ultimate meaning of physical illness. He starts with the nature of personhood, and how illness has come "to be construed as uniquely physiological and somehow independent of the afflicted person." He considers the harm we do others by refusing to consider the spiritual dimension of human persons. He has a "must-read" chapter on the spiritual meaning of illness. Finally, he looks at Christian paths toward healing. He reminds us that the early church fathers did not regard Christ as either a "Physician of bodies," or, a "Physician of souls." They most frequently called Him by the title "Physician of the soul and body."

Paul Tournier, *A Doctor's Casebook in Light of the Bible* (Harper and Row, Publishers, 1954)

By the author of "The Meaning of Persons," this is a delightful book describing many of Dr. Tournier's patient cases, connecting medicine and ministry. "We may say, then, that every illness calls for two diagnoses: one scientific, nosological and causal, and the other spiritual, a diagnosis of its meaning and purpose," explaining that the first is made by the doctor and the second made by the patient. He says, "From the point of view of the patient's eternal destiny, the second diagnosis is much more important than the first."

Kuhn, W.T., *Heal in Imitation of Christ: Conversations on Medical Missions* **(Trusted Books, 2014)**

A helpful guide to the many questions students ask about medical missions, from preparation to practice. Written by a modern physician, who served with his wife, also a doctor, in Asia, and continues to be involved in mentoring others.

Shelly, Judith Allen; Miller, Arlene B.; and Fenstermacher, Kimberly, H., *Called to Care: A Christian Vision for Nursing* **(Inter-Varsity Press, 2021, Third edition)**

The authors say, "This book is addressed primarily to nurses who call themselves Christian and are trying to think through the implications of that commitment in their professional lives." They demonstrate how a Christian worldview can be distorted by other cultural worldviews. They look not just at the theory of nursing but the theology of nursing, showing how true nursing cannot be divorced from the Christian story. They define Christian nursing as "a ministry of compassionate care for the whole person, in response to God's grace toward a sinful world, which aims to foster optimum health (*shalom*) and bring comfort in suffering and death for anyone in need."

Allberry, Sam., *What God Has to Say about Our Bodies: How the Gospel is Good News for Our Physical Selves* **(Wheaton: Crossway Books, 2021)**

This little book brings the body back into discipleship. "A gospel for souls that excludes or overlooks our bodies is not the gospel of Scripture. The gospel without a theology of the body is a truncated, inadequate gospel. A church that doesn't have a robust gospel theology of the body will be unprepared to meet this generation's philosophical, psychological, sociological, scientific, and media challenges." This is a gentle, pastoral approach, not an academic one.

Cutillo, Bob, *Pursuing Health in an Anxious Age* (Wheaton, Illinois: Crossway, 2016)

The author helps us cultivate a biblical understanding of faith and health for the modern age. He quotes the proverb, "The corruption of the best is the worst," showing how the good gift of health has been corrupted. He challenges the cultural idea that we can flourish on our own terms rather than God's. He says that modern medicine is like a river that has overflowed its boundaries and wants us to help medicine understand its proper place. Highly recommended.

* * *

The work of God through history and mission

Stark, R., *The Rise of Christianity: How the Obscure, Marginal Jesus Movement Became the Dominant Religious Force in the Western World in a Few Centuries* (San Francisco: Harper One, 1996)

Rodney Stark is a sociologist writing a persuasive account of how Christianity became dominant in the Roman Empire and has changed the Western world. Chapter 4 (Epidemics, Networks and Conversion) details the response of Christians to the tragic epidemics of the time, and the resulting side effect: the growth of the church.

Ferngren, G.B., *Medicine and Health Care in Early Christianity* (Baltimore: Johns Hopkins University Press, 2009)

Written by a historian, this academic work explores the attitudes of early Christians to medicine and physicians. He explains how the erroneous assumption that Christians were opposed to medicine became popular. He counteracts that popular assumption with evidence that Christians engaged in natural means of healing just like others in their world, rather than attributing most diseases to demons or seeking miraculous cures. "The fact that the naturalistic basis of medicine was value-neutral made it relatively benign in religious terms." Here are important lessons for us as modern Christians, as we seek to integrate the natural with the spiritual.

Walls, A.F., *The Missionary Movement in Christian History* (Maryknoll, New York: Orbis Books, 2005)

Walls is a missiologist who explores the role of the Christian culture of the West in the missionary movement. He helps move us beyond missions as only "from the West to the rest" to a more global exchange from one culture to another. While the Gospel of Jesus Christ remains central to our mission task, it does not produce a single "true" Christian culture. Rather, it transforms every culture of the world. To transform cultures, medical or healthcare missionaries must increasingly represent a diversity of cultures. Healthcare professionals serving across cultures have much to learn from these missiological conversations.

Grundmann, C.H., *Sent to Heal! Emergence and Development of Medical Missions* (Lanham: University Press of America, 2005)

This is a must-read for medical professionals in missions. Grundmann, a Professor of Theology and friend of the medical mission enterprise traces the roots of the enterprise from the early days of William Carey in the 1790s. He describes how the concept (and label) of "medical missions" came about and gained legitimacy in the 19th century as a full-fledged member of the mission enterprise. He unpacks medical professionals' challenges in defining and defending the work to mission leaders. An indispensable guide, especially to the first period of medical missions, ending in the late 20th century.

Bryant Myers, Erin Dufault-Hunter and Issac Voss Health, *Healing and Shalom: Frontiers and Challenges for Christian Health Missions* (William Carey Library, 2015)

This book argues that Christians should reclaim their legacy of influence in healthcare. The authors write, "Do our efforts reflect a firm and substantial theological foundation or are we just baptizing modern Western Medicine with some Bible verses and prayers, as Dr. Dan Fountain wonders in this volume?" It outlines approaches to "putting the whole person back together." Centered on the theme of *shalom*, the editors want to motivate us to extend and build upon health systems and services to the poor through biblically-based approaches. They especially want to reawaken the church to the centrality of health and wholeness in the mission of Christ.

Leadership

Blackaby, H. and Blackaby, R., *Spiritual Leadership* (Nashville: Broadman and Holman, 2001)

A classic work in which the Blackabys help us look beyond tasks and results to something deeper. "The primary goal of spiritual leadership is not excellence, in the sense of doing things perfectly. Rather, it is taking people from where they are to where God wants them to be." They emphasize that God uses relationships and events to grow amateurs into leaders, not wasting any experiences. This work can help you embrace leadership without fear since Christ is at work within you.

Sherman, A.L., *Kingdom Calling: Vocational Stewardship for the Common Good* (Downers Grove: IV Press, 2011)

The book is about integrating faith and work. Sherman writes for any vocation, not just medical professionals. But her treatment of "righteousness" and its implications for justice are pertinent to our conversation about the community outside the hospital or clinic. Her research shows that many evangelicals perch atop their career ladders in various social circles but with a "profoundly anemic vision for what they could accomplish for the Kingdom of God." She begins by sharing Tim Keller's definition of the righteous, as those "willing to disadvantage themselves for the community while the wicked are those who put their own economic, social, and personal needs ahead of the needs of the community." We need to have conversations about vocational stewardship for the common good together with disciples and churches we partner with.

Kelly M. Kapic, *You're Only Human: How Your Limits Reflect God's Design and Why That's Good News* **(Brazos Press, 2022)**

A simple and practical approach to living within the limits that God has given us, and how these limits may themselves be a gift from God. Kapic wants to relieve us from the burden of trying to be something we are not and cannot be.

Lingenfelter, S.G., *Leadership in the Way of the Cross: Forging Ministry from the Crucible of Crisis* **(Cascade Books, 2018)**

The author speaks from his long experience as an academic leader. He shares his failures with us and demonstrates how vulnerability is key to effective leadership. Our default leadership patterns are often driven by fear of failure or a quest for significance. He demonstrates how God can use conflict to draw out these deep fears and "hungers," shaping us as servants rather than leaders who must command and control. He helps us move beyond our concern for ministry performance to God's concern that we become His covenant people.

APPENDIX C

Selected Definitions

Corruption: The process by which something is changed from its original use or meaning to something erroneous or debased. Sin does not make us unhuman, but corrupts our entire personhood, orienting us away from God's authority and direction.

Cultural mandate: The cultural mandate is like a basic job description for humanity. Human beings are to work under God for the sake of human flourishing. We are designed for connections with others to fulfill God's will for others.

Design: An inherent plan that unfolds because of the way something is created. There is a design, or purpose, in individual created things, but there is also a larger, grand design, for the whole of creation. That grand design gives meaning and purpose to our work in healthcare ministry.

Selected Definitions

Disciple-making: Inviting others to know Jesus and make Him known. Making disciples fulfills Christ's Great Commission by enabling others to fulfill God's cultural mandate to love God and neighbor. Thus it is the core ministry goal of both healthcare ministry and mission.

Fall: The Fall was the event that ushered sin into the world, "a radical disruption of the core of our being."[195]

Gospel: The good news of redemption through Christ, by which He saves us from sin (by His own death, thus changing the direction of our lives toward God) and for righteousness (by giving us His new life). Redemption is both personal and corporate since Christ gives us new bodies and places us together in His own body, the church. Jesus continues to bring the gospel to the afflicted and to bind up the brokenhearted (Isaiah 61:1) through the church. We join Him by living the life and speaking the words He has given us.

Health: A state of integrated physical and spiritual well-being, which Scripture declares to be possible ultimately only through faith in Jesus Christ. Healing is the restoration of that well-being by God's gracious work.

Healthcare: Human effort to relieve the suffering of others through the organized provision of medical care. More broadly, it can extend to efforts to control disease and promote health.

---

[195] Frame, *Systematic Theology*, 850.

Healthcare ministry: Christian healthcare, motivated by the compassion and example of Jesus. Healthcare ministry proclaims the gospel in word and deed as a service to the whole person and community, making disciples of Jesus in the process.

Healthcare mission: The work of God through healthcare ministry, usually in partnership with other ministries such as church planting and evangelism. The mission of healthcare is not about compassionate medical care alone but has the whole mission of God in view. Healthcare is anchored in the wider mission of God by making disciples.

Kingdom of God: The Kingdom of God is one way Scripture describes how God is carrying about His purpose in the world. The Kingdom is present in the world (now) and also a future reality (not yet).

Medical mission: I have used this term to refer to the first century and a half of the Protestant mission to the world (approximately 1830-1970), born out of the twin motivations of scientific advances and world evangelization. More broadly today, medical mission can refer to the clinical component of healthcare mission.

Ministry: Service to mankind for the glory of God, even in the face of opposition. Ministry is obedience to Jesus in everything. It encompasses evangelism (proclaiming the gospel) and goes beyond it to disciple-making and church planting. Ministry is anchored in the mission of God.

Selected Definitions

Mission of God: The work of God in the world, in history, to redeem human beings from sin and bring about a new creation in Christ. God accomplishes this mission through the church but His purpose goes beyond the church and extends to the entire world, restoring creation. I sometimes use simply "mission" to refer to the big picture of God's work, and "ministry" to refer to components or strategies within the mission of God.

Person: A human being made in God's image to be an unbroken reflection of God to creation. A unique individual, made for that purpose out of things material and immaterial. A social creature, made to be in a relationship with others for God's glory. Created as male and female to serve together.

Salvation (redemption): Salvation is whole-person healing. The Old Testament uses the Hebrew word for salvation as deliverance from military victory or danger in general. The New Testament word for salvation means not only health, safety, and deliverance from danger but also deliverance from the penalty and power of sin. In both Testaments, salvation is holistic and involves the whole person's well-being, not just his mind or spirit.

Shalom: The Hebrew term for peace, reconciliation, and harmony which flows from a right relationship with God and others. *Shalom* is a characteristic of the Kingdom of God. As we work toward *shalom* through healthcare ministry, we also recognize that there are spiritual forces opposing *shalom* and the Kingdom of God, and thus healthcare ministry is also a spiritual battle against these forces.

Soul: The soul is a person from the spiritual point of view, designed to worship and obey God. The soul is made from the breath of God for meaning and purpose. The body, on the other hand, is a person from a material point of view, made from the dust of the earth. Soul and body are an integrated whole.

Worldview: The mental map, framework, or design that makes sense of our lives and gives meaning. It can also be understood as the big story we are part of, helping us understand who we are, what went wrong, and how we must respond.

Acknowledgments

I used to think a book was written by its author. Now I realize it is a team sport. You would not be holding this book without the inspiration and support of others.

My Dad, a New York Times reporter and lifelong storyteller, taught me to think before writing. He also helped me understand that writing is not "all about me." Dad passed away just as I finished this manuscript, at 98. Thank you, Dad, for your legacy.

Clare, you helped me illustrate the stories and experiences we shared in three decades of ministry together in Ethiopia, Nepal, Thailand, and beyond. And you gave me the gift of working with me through more edits than I can count. Thank you, Beth, John, Amy, and Hannah. As children, you embraced the ups and downs of missionary life on three continents; as adults, you have made us proud!

There is a special place in my heart for you, Ato Mardikios, for your patience with me as a green and impatient first-term missionary in Arba Minch, Ethiopia. As an Ethiopian church leader and friend, you helped me learn from those I had come to serve. You also warned me not to "overthink." May God bless you for your

Acknowledgments

faithful life of service to our Lord Jesus Christ as a father, a pharmacist, and a church elder.

As friends and fellow authors, Gary Corwin and John Sittema encouraged me to put down my thoughts on paper and supported me in the writing process. My SIM Health Ministry Team gave me the time to complete it. It is a privilege to "shape, support, and strengthen" SIM health ministries with you, friends: Kendrick Lau, Bob Blees, Quinton Friesen, John Barnshaw, Dave and Margie Burgess, Phil Andrew, Mark and Jana Faus, Beth Roberts, Ann-Britt Smazik and Sue Penno.

I cannot begin to mention countless individuals who have mentored, coached, and shaped me. I am so grateful for our years with SIM and the people who have made my life richer, from leaders to teammates to healthcare missionaries. I bless the Lord for a friendship with Dr. Ken Gamble of Missionary Health Institute in Toronto, who helped me better care for the whole-person needs of missionaries, including mental health and resilience. I am grateful for church and mission leaders from various denominations and agencies around the world who have modeled Christ to me. Your lives have inspired me to love others as Jesus did. May He lift each of you with wings like an eagle.

I have been helped by a community of creators and teachers of "Christian Global Health in Perspective," an online course under Health for All Nations. Course students (African and Asian healthcare professionals) have helped inspire some of the work. It has been great to work with you on this course: Mike Soderling, Dan O'Neill, Christoffer Grundmann, Neil Thompson, Bruce Dahlman, Perry Jansen, Rebecca Myer, and Jason Lee.

As my editor, Andy Richards, you have been a cheerleader, encouraging me to stay the course and helping with many practical details. You have been a blessing. Your editing, too, was just what I needed, Megan Tatreau. Thank you, Jan Cox; not many sisters-in-law could help me improve my copy and find all those comma splices! I'm also grateful to you, Jeannette Taylor, for your sage marketing guidance. Friends at Genesis Publishing, your excellent work has helped make the dream a reality.

Elisabeth Kvernen and Hannah Hudson, you encouraged your Dad during the writing and the design. Who would have thought a cover design and layout was so important? You kept me on track. And Chelsea Hudson, thanks for your advice and photos!

I am grateful to you who critiqued drafts and made the book stronger: Gary Corwin, John Sittema, Dan O'Neill, Stan Key, Dave and Margie Burgess, Niles and Rachel Batdorf, Tim Teusink, Neil Thompson, Jarry Richardson, Christoffer Grundmann, Mark and Jana Faus, Quinton Friesen. A special thanks to Dr. Dan O'Neill and Christoffer Grundmann, who patiently reviewed every page!

Lord Jesus, I praise you for your life, love, and forgiveness. Your Word has brought contentment and joy.

If you found this book helpful, will you consider sharing the message with others by posting a review on a retail website or social media? I would so appreciate your help in spreading the word about *Healthcare and the Mission of God*.

In addition, I'd love to hear from you. Feel free to contact me at paul@pauljhudson.com. You can also learn more of my story and read updated postings at pauljhudson.com.